ENZO MILANO

DIABETES

CAUSES, DIAGNOSIS, AND MANAGEMENT

Includes Exercise and Nutrition Planners, and Self-Check Record Template

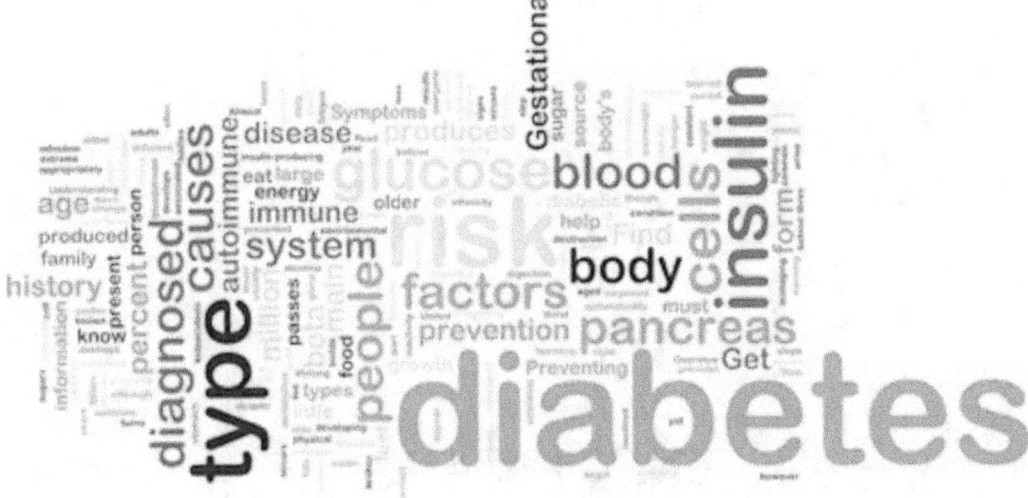

DIABETES

Causes, Diagnosis, and Management

ENZO MILANO

RED DOT PUBLICATIONS ©

Table of Contents

Introduction

Living with diabetes requires a delicate balance between various aspects of life. It's crucial to strike a balance between diet, physical activity, and medication to effectively manage the condition. However, managing diabetes isn't just about finding the right balance between these elements. It's also about maintaining a balance in other areas of life, such as work, relationships, and mental health.

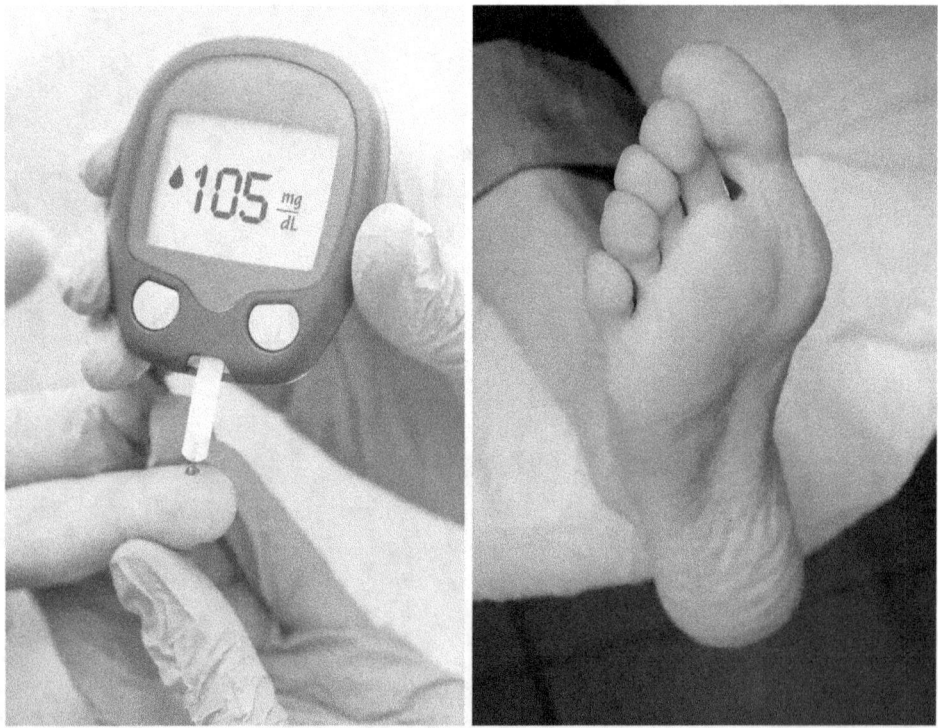

Finding the right balance can be challenging, but it's not impossible. With the support of loved ones, healthcare professionals, and the community, individuals with diabetes can take charge of their condition and live a healthy, fulfilling life. Remember that diabetes is a lifelong condition, and managing it requires a long-term commitment to healthy habits and self-care.

Achieving balance in life with diabetes involves making healthy lifestyle choices, such as following a balanced diet, engaging in regular physical activity, and adhering to a medication regimen. It's also important to prioritize mental health and well-being, as stress and anxiety can have a negative impact on diabetes management.

In addition to individual efforts, it's necessary to have a strong support system. Family and friends can provide emotional support and encouragement, while healthcare professionals can offer guidance and advice on managing diabetes. The community can also play a role in supporting individuals with diabetes by promoting healthy living initiatives and providing resources for diabetes management.

Ultimately, living well with diabetes requires a multifaceted approach that incorporates balance in all aspects of life. By finding the right balance between diet, physical activity, medication, work, relationships, and mental health, individuals with diabetes can take charge of their condition and live a healthy, fulfilling life.

What Is Diabetes?

Diabetes is a condition where the body has difficulty regulating blood sugar levels. Normally, the pancreas produces insulin, a hormone that helps glucose (sugar) from food enter the body's cells for energy. In diabetes, the body either doesn't produce enough insulin or can't use its own insulin effectively, leading to high levels of glucose building up in the blood.

There are two main types of diabetes

- Type 1 diabetes: In this type, the body doesn't produce enough insulin, usually because the immune system mistakenly attacks and destroys the cells in the pancreas that produce insulin. Type 1 diabetes typically develops in childhood or adolescence, and people with this condition need to take insulin injections to control their blood sugar levels.

- Type 2 diabetes: In this type, the body can't use its own insulin effectively, often due to factors such as being overweight or inactive. Type 2 diabetes is the most common form of diabetes and can often be managed through lifestyle changes, such as eating a healthy diet and exercising regularly.

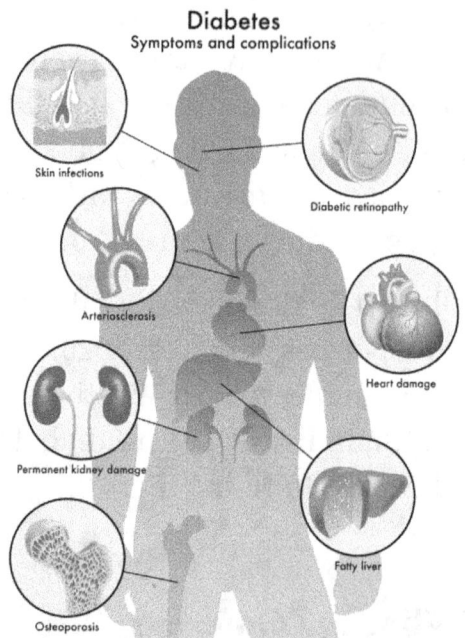

If left untreated, diabetes can lead to a range of complications, including:

* Heart disease and stroke

* Kidney damage

* Nerve damage

* Eye damage, including blindness

* Infections and poor wound healing

Fortunately, with proper management, people with diabetes can lead long and healthy lives. This involves monitoring blood sugar levels, following a healthy diet, getting regular exercise, and taking medications as needed.

Signs and Symptoms of Diabetes

Diabetes is a serious medical condition that can have significant consequences if left untreated. It's relevant for individuals to be aware of the signs and symptoms of diabetes, so they can seek medical attention if they suspect they may have the condition. In this response, we'll explore the signs and symptoms of diabetes in more detail, including the effects of high blood sugar levels on the body.

Here are the signs and symptoms of diabetes:

- Increased thirst and hunger: When there's too much glucose in the blood, the body tries to flush it out by producing more urine, which can lead to dehydration. This can cause feelings of thirst that don't go away even after drinking plenty of water. Additionally, high blood sugar levels can cause an increase in hunger, as the body tries to burn more energy to compensate for the excess glucose.

- Frequent urination: With high levels of glucose in the blood, the kidneys will try to flush it out by producing more urine, leading to frequent trips to the bathroom. This can be especially noticeable at night, when it may disrupt sleep patterns.

- Blurry vision: High blood sugar levels can cause the lens in the eye to swell, leading to blurry vision. This can make it difficult to focus on objects, read, or drive.

- Fatigue: When the body is unable to properly use glucose for energy, it can lead to feelings of fatigue. This can be especially pronounced after eating a meal that causes a spike in blood sugar levels.

- Weight loss: Even though the body is not able to properly use glucose for energy, it may still try to burn fat for energy, leading to weight loss. This can be especially noticeable in the face, arms, and legs.

- Dry skin: High blood sugar levels can cause dry skin, which can lead to itchiness and irritation. This can be especially noticeable in areas like the hands, feet, and legs.

- Sores that don't heal: High blood sugar levels can affect the body's ability to heal wounds, which can lead to sores that don't heal properly. This can be especially concerning for people with diabetes, as it can lead to infections and other complications.

- Frequent infections: High blood sugar levels can weaken the immune system, making it easier for infections to occur. This can include urinary tract infections, yeast infections, and other types of infections.

- Numbness or tingling in the feet: High blood sugar levels can damage the nerves, leading to numbness or tingling sensations in the feet and legs. This can be especially concerning, as it can lead to injuries or other complications if left untreated.

- Vomiting: In some cases, people with diabetes may experience vomiting, especially if they have high blood sugar levels or are experiencing a severe hypoglycemic episode.

Note that not everyone with diabetes will experience all of these symptoms, and some people may not experience any symptoms at all. However, if you do experience any of these symptoms, be sure to speak with your healthcare provider to determine the cause and appropriate treatment.

Types of Diabetes

I. Type 1 Diabetes

* Definition: Type 1 diabetes is a chronic autoimmune disease in which the pancreas produces little or no insulin, a hormone that regulates blood sugar levels.

* Symptoms: Symptoms of type 1 diabetes can develop quickly, often over the course of a few weeks, and may include increased thirst and urination, fatigue, weight loss, and blurred vision.

* Causes: Type 1 diabetes is caused by the immune system attacking and destroying the cells in the pancreas that produce insulin, resulting in a complete deficiency of insulin production.

* Treatment: People with type 1 diabetes must inject insulin daily to manage their blood sugar levels. They must also monitor their blood sugar levels regularly and make adjustments to their insulin doses based on their food intake, physical activity, and other factors.

II. Type 2 Diabetes

* Definition: Type 2 diabetes is a chronic condition that affects the way the body regulates blood sugar levels. It is caused by a combination of insulin resistance (when the body's cells become less responsive to insulin) and impaired insulin secretion.

* Symptoms: Symptoms of type 2 diabetes can develop gradually over time and

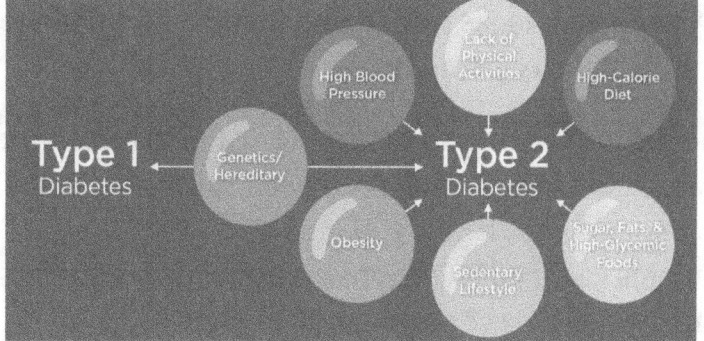

may include increased thirst and urination, fatigue, weight loss, and blurred vision.

* Causes: Type 2 diabetes is caused by a combination of genetic and lifestyle factors, including obesity, physical inactivity, and an unhealthy diet.

* Treatment: Treatment for type 2 diabetes typically involves a combination of lifestyle changes, such as a healthy diet and regular exercise, as well as medication to help manage blood sugar levels. In some cases, insulin therapy may be necessary.

There are also other types of diabetes, such as gestational diabetes (which occurs during pregnancy) and LADA (latent autoimmune diabetes in adults), as well as prediabetes (a condition in which blood sugar levels are higher than normal but not high enough to be classified as diabetes).

Type 2 diabetes is the most common form of diabetes, accounting for approximately 90% of all diabetes cases. It is a metabolic disorder that affects the way the body regulates blood sugar levels. In type 2 diabetes, the pancreas continues to produce insulin, but the body's cells become less responsive to it, leading to high blood sugar levels.

Type 2 diabetes is often associated with older age, obesity, physical inactivity, and a family history of diabetes. However, in recent years, there has been an increase in the number of children and young adults being diagnosed with type 2 diabetes. This is thought to be due to a combination of factors, including the rising prevalence of obesity and physical inactivity in young people, as well as the increasing incidence of type 2 diabetes in ethnic minority populations.

The symptoms of type 2 diabetes can be subtle and may develop gradually over time. They include increased thirst and urination, fatigue, blurred vision, and slow healing of cuts and wounds. If left untreated, type 2 diabetes can lead to serious complications, such as heart disease, kidney damage, and nerve damage.

Fortunately, type 2 diabetes can often be managed through lifestyle changes, such as a healthy diet and regular physical activity. Medications, including metformin, can also be used to help control blood sugar levels. In some cases, insulin therapy may be necessary.

Early detection and treatment of type 2 diabetes are important for preventing long-term complications. If you have any concerns about your risk for type 2 diabetes or are experiencing symptoms, it is important to speak with your healthcare provider. They can help determine your risk and develop a plan to manage your diabetes.

Type 2 diabetes is a common form of diabetes that affects the way the body regulates blood sugar levels. It is often associated with older age, obesity, physical inactivity, and a family history of diabetes. However, it can also occur in children and young adults, particularly in those who are overweight or have a family history of diabetes. Early detection and treatment are important for preventing long-term complications.

Risk factors for developing type 2 diabetes

- Family history: Having a first-degree relative (such as a parent or sibling) with diabetes increases your risk of developing the disease.

- Lack of physical activity: A sedentary lifestyle can increase your risk of developing type 2 diabetes.

- Overweight or obesity: Being overweight or obese is a major risk factor for developing type 2 diabetes, as excess body fat can increase resistance to insulin.

- Unhealthy diet: Consuming a diet high in processed foods, sugar, and saturated fats can increase your risk of developing type 2 diabetes.

- Ethnicity: Certain ethnic groups, such as Asian, Pacific Islander, Native Hawaiian, American Indian, Hispanic, Latino, or African American, have a higher risk of developing type 2 diabetes.

- Age: The risk of developing type 2 diabetes increases with age, especially after the age of 4 -

- Gestational diabetes: Women who have had gestational diabetes during pregnancy are at a higher risk of developing type 2 diabetes later in life.

- Polycystic ovary syndrome (PCOS): Women with PCOS are at a higher risk of developing insulin resistance and type 2 diabetes.

- Sleep apnea: People with sleep apnea are at a higher risk of developing type 2 diabetes, as sleep apnea can disrupt normal sleep patterns and increase inflammation in the body.

- Certain medications: Some medications, such as corticosteroids and certain antipsychotic drugs, can increase the risk of developing type 2 diabetes.

Not everyone with these risk factors will develop type 2 diabetes, and some people may develop the disease without any known risk factors. If you're concerned about your risk of developing type 2 diabetes, talk to your doctor about your individual risk factors and what you can do to reduce your risk.

Diabetes Control

Diet

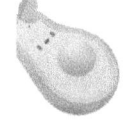

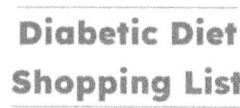

Diabetic Diet Shopping List

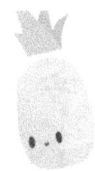

Eat Three Meals a Day

A. Diet

Vegetables
○ Broccoli
○ Spinach
○ Kale
○ Cauliflower
○ Brussels sprouts
○ Asparagus
○ Cucumbers
○ Bell peppers
○ Zucchini
○ Mushrooms

Protein Sources
○ Chicken breast
○ Turkey
○ Fish (salmon, tuna, mackerel)
○ Tofu
○ Eggs
○ Cottage cheese (low-fat or fat-free)
○ Greek yogurt (unsweetened)

Whole Grains
○ Oats
○ Quinoa
○ Brown rice
○ Whole wheat bread
○ Barley
○ Bulgur

Legumes
○ Lentils
○ Chickpeas
○ Black beans
○ Kidney beans

Healthy Fat
○ Olive oil
○ Avocado oil
○ Almonds
○ Walnuts
○ Chia seeds
○ Flaxseeds
○ Pumpkin seeds
○ Nut butter (almond, peanut, cashew)

Fruit
○ Berries (blueberries, strawberries, raspberries)
○ Citrus fruits
○ Avocado
○ Apples
○ Pears
○ Peaches
○ Plums
○ Kiwi
○ Grapes
○ Watermelon
○ Pineapple
○ Mango

Dairy Alternatives
○ Unsweetened almond milk
○ Unsweetened coconut milk
○ Unsweetened soy milk

Diet plays a crucial role in diabetes control. The food we eat affects our blood sugar levels, and a healthy diet can help manage diabetes by maintaining healthy blood sugar levels, achieving a healthy body weight, and providing the body with the necessary nutrients to function properly.

- Maintaining healthy blood sugar levels:

The primary goal of a diabetes diet is to maintain healthy blood sugar levels. This can be achieved by consuming foods that are low in sugar, refined carbohydrates, and saturated fats. A healthy diet should include plenty of fruits, vegetables, whole grains, lean protein sources, and healthy fats. These foods are rich in fiber, vitamins, minerals, and antioxidants that help regulate blood sugar levels and improve insulin sensitivity.

- Maintaining or achieving healthy body weight:

A healthy diet can also help individuals with diabetes maintain or achieve a healthy body weight. Excess weight can increase insulin resistance, making it harder to manage blood sugar levels. A diet rich in nutrient-dense foods and low in calories can help promote weight loss and improve health.

- Eating the right amount of healthy foods:

The amount of food we eat is also important in diabetes control. Eating too much food can lead to high blood sugar levels, while eating too little food can lead to low blood sugar levels. A healthy diet should include the right amount of food to maintain healthy blood sugar levels and provide the body with the necessary nutrients.

In addition to the above goals, a healthy diet can also help individuals with diabetes manage their medication and insulin doses, reduce the risk of complications, and improve their quality of life.

A healthy diet is not a one-size-fits-all approach. A registered dietitian or a healthcare provider can help individuals with diabetes develop a personalized meal plan that takes into account their specific needs, lifestyle, and health goals.

- Eat Three Meals a Day

Eating at least three meals a day is an important aspect of maintaining healthy blood sugar levels. Skipping meals or going too long without eating can lead to low blood sugar, which can cause a range of symptoms including dizziness, fatigue, and irritability. Eating regular meals can also help prevent high blood sugar, which can damage organs and tissues over time.

The American Diabetes Association recommends that individuals with diabetes aim to eat at least three meals a day, with healthy snacks in between meals as needed. This can help keep blood sugar levels stable and prevent large spikes in blood sugar that can occur after skipping meals.

In addition to eating three meals a day, some individuals with diabetes may also benefit from having 5-6 smaller meals throughout the day. This approach can help keep blood sugar levels stable and prevent large spikes in blood sugar that can occur after eating large meals. However, keep in mind that this approach may not be suitable for everyone, and it's best to consult with a healthcare provider or registered dietitian to determine the best meal plan for your individual needs.

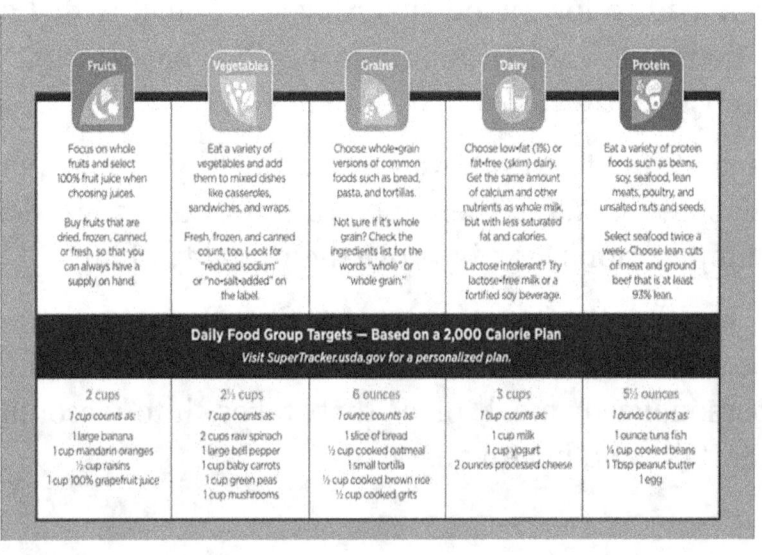

Healthy snacks can also play an important role in maintaining healthy blood sugar levels. Snacks can help prevent low blood sugar and provide additional nutrients and energy throughout the day. Some healthy snack options include fruits, vegetables, nuts, seeds, and low-fat dairy products. Choose snacks that are low in added sugars, saturated fats, and sodium, and high in fiber and nutrients.

Eating at least three meals a day with healthy snacks in between can help maintain healthy blood sugar levels and prevent complications associated with diabetes. Consult with a healthcare provider or registered dietitian to determine the best meal plan for your individual needs.

Pay Attention to Food Portions

Paying attention to food portions is a crucial aspect of managing blood sugar levels. Consuming large portions of food can lead to consuming more calories, carbohydrates, and added sugars than needed, which can cause blood sugar levels to spike. This can be particularly challenging for individuals with diabetes, as their bodies may have difficulty regulating blood sugar levels.

To control blood sugar levels, it's essential to limit food portions and consume only the recommended amount of food at each meal. This can help prevent large spikes in blood sugar and keep levels within a healthy range.

Here are some tips for paying attention to food portions:

 - Use measuring cups or a food scale to measure out the recommended portion size of each food item.

 - Choose smaller plates to help control portion sizes and prevent overeating.

 - Eat slowly and savor your food to help you feel full and satisfied before consuming large portions.

 - Avoid eating in front of screens, such as the TV or computer, as it can lead to mindless snacking and overeating.

 - Be aware of portion sizes when eating out and choose menu items that are lower in calories and carbohydrates.

 - Consider sharing meals or taking home leftovers for another meal to avoid overeating.

Paying attention to food portions is a crucial aspect of managing blood sugar levels. Consuming large portions of food can lead to consuming more calories, carbohydrates, and added sugars than needed, which can cause blood sugar levels to spike. This can be particularly challenging for individuals with diabetes, as their bodies may have difficulty regulating blood sugar levels.

To control blood sugar levels, it's essential to limit food portions and consume only the recommended amount of food at each meal. This can help prevent large spikes in blood sugar and keep levels within a healthy range.

Here are some tips for paying attention to food portions:

- Use measuring cups or a food scale to measure out the recommended portion size of each food item.

- Choose smaller plates to help control portion sizes and prevent overeating.

- Eat slowly and savor your food to help you feel full and satisfied before consuming large portions.

- Avoid eating in front of screens, such as the TV or computer, as it can lead to mindless snacking and overeating.

- Be aware of portion sizes when eating out and choose menu items that are lower in calories and carbohydrates.

- Consider sharing meals or taking home leftovers for another meal to avoid overeating.

By paying attention to food portions, individuals with diabetes can better manage their blood sugar levels and prevent complications associated with the disease. Consult with a healthcare provider or registered dietitian to determine the appropriate portion sizes and develop a personalized meal plan.

Choose Foods From Three or More Food Groups for Each Meal

When it comes to managing blood sugar levels, it's crucial to eat a balanced diet that includes a variety of foods from different food groups. By choosing foods from three or more food groups for each meal, you can help keep your blood sugar levels within a healthy range.

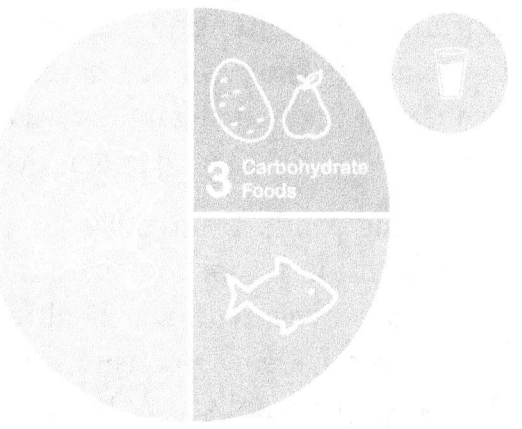

The reason for this is that different food groups provide different nutrients and energy sources that can help regulate blood sugar levels. For example:

- Starches: Starches, such as whole grains, fruits, and vegetables, provide carbohydrates, which are broken down into glucose and used as energy.

- Protein: Protein, such as lean meats, poultry, fish, and legumes, helps to slow down the digestion of carbohydrates and can help regulate blood sugar levels.

- Vegetables: Vegetables, such as leafy greens, broccoli, and bell peppers, provide fiber, vitamins, and minerals that can help regulate blood sugar levels and improve health.

By combining foods from these groups, you can create a balanced meal that provides a steady source of energy and helps to regulate blood sugar levels. For example, a meal that includes a starch, such as brown rice, a protein, such as grilled chicken, and a vegetable, such as steamed broccoli, can help keep blood sugar levels within a healthy range.

In addition to choosing foods from three or more food groups, it's also important to pay attention to portion sizes and the quality of the foods you eat. Choosing whole, unprocessed foods whenever possible and limiting your intake of added sugars, saturated fats, and refined carbohydrates can also help to regulate blood sugar levels and improve health.

By choosing foods from three or more food groups for each meal and paying attention to portion sizes and food quality, you can help keep your blood sugar levels within a healthy range and improve your health. It's always a good idea to consult with a healthcare provider or registered dietitian for personalized nutrition advice and to develop a meal plan that meets your individual needs.

Choose Foods Lower in Fat

Tips for choosing foods lower in fat:

 - Opt for baked, grilled, or roasted foods instead of fried foods.

 - Use herbs and spices to add flavor to your food instead of relying on butter or margarine.

 - Choose lean protein sources like chicken, fish, and tofu instead of high-fat meats like sausage and bacon.

 - Limit your intake of canned meats, pre-packaged foods, and other processed foods that are high in fat.

 - Use olive oil or avocado oil instead of coconut oil or lard for cooking.

- Avoid mayonnaise and other high-fat condiments like soy sauce and teriyaki sauce.

- Choose low-fat dairy products like skim milk, Greek yogurt, and cottage cheese instead of full-fat dairy products.

- Snack on fruits, vegetables, and nuts instead of high-fat snacks like chips and crackers.

- Be mindful of portion sizes and don't consume too many calories.

- Read food labels and choose products that are low in fat and added sugars.

Remember to maintain a balanced diet and consume some healthy fats for energy and nutrition. However, by limiting your intake of high-fat foods and choosing lower-fat options, you can help reduce your risk of heart disease and maintain a healthy weight.

Choose Foods High in Fiber

Tips for choosing foods high in fiber:

- Opt for whole grains like brown rice, quinoa, and whole wheat bread instead of refined grains like white rice and white bread.

- Incorporate more beans into your diet, such as black beans, kidney beans, and chickpeas.

- Eat a variety of fresh vegetables and fruits, such as broccoli, carrots, apples, and berries.

- Snack on nuts and seeds like almonds, pumpkin seeds, and chia seeds.

- Choose high-fiber cereals like oatmeal or bran cereal for breakfast.

- Incorporate more whole grains like barley, farro, and bulgur into your meals.

- Try incorporating some high-fiber foods into your smoothies or juices, such as spinach, kale, or flaxseeds.

- Choose whole grain pasta instead of refined pasta.

- Try some new high-fiber foods like psyllium husk or ground flaxseeds.

- Read food labels and choose products that are high in fiber.

Remember to increase your fiber intake gradually to allow your body to adjust. Aim to consume at least 25 grams of fiber per day for women and 38 grams per day for men. High-fiber foods can help promote digestive health, lower cholesterol levels, and support healthy blood sugar levels.

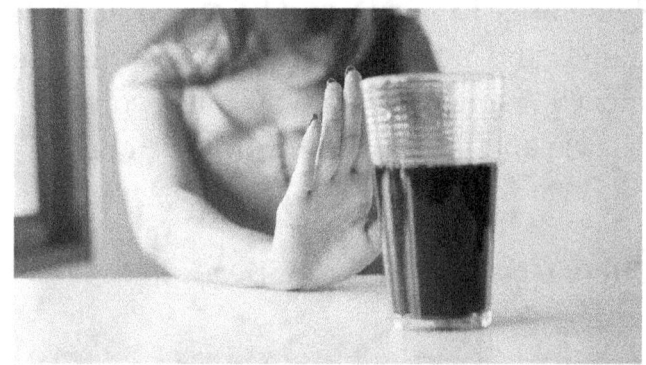

Limit Sweets and Alcohol

Tips for limiting sweets and alcohol:

- Read food labels: Check the ingredient list and nutrition facts panel to see if a food contains added sugars. Look for hidden sources of sugar, such as high fructose corn syrup, agave nectar, or honey.

- Choose unsweetened products: Opt for unsweetened yogurt, almond milk, and other dairy alternatives. Select unsweetened applesauce, canned fruit, and other packaged foods.

- Limit portion sizes: Enjoy sweets and alcohol in moderation. Choose smaller portions or share a dessert with a friend.

- Eat sweets after meals: Eating sweets after meals can help reduce the spike in blood sugar levels.

- Avoid sugary drinks: Sugary drinks, like soda and sports drinks, are high in added sugars and can quickly add up. Opt for water, unsweetened tea, or black coffee instead.

- Be mindful of alcohol intake: Limit alcohol intake to moderate levels (up to one drink per day for women and up to two drinks per day for men). Excessive alcohol consumption can raise blood sugar levels and increase the risk of health complications.

- Choose low-alcohol drinks: Opt for drinks with lower alcohol content, such as beer or wine, instead of high-alcohol cocktails or shots.

- Eat before or while drinking: Eating before or while drinking can help slow down the absorption of alcohol into the bloodstream, which can help reduce the impact on blood sugar levels.

- Monitor your blood sugar levels: If you have diabetes, monitor your blood sugar levels regularly to ensure that your levels remain within a healthy range. Adjust your diet and physical activity accordingly.

- Seek support: If you're struggling to limit sweets and alcohol, consider seeking support from a registered dietitian or a certified diabetes educator. They can help you develop a personalized meal plan and provide guidance on managing blood sugar levels.

Work with your healthcare provider to determine the best approaches for managing your blood sugar levels. They can provide personalized advice and help you develop a plan that's tailored to your individual needs.

Physical Activity

Physical activity is a crucial component of managing diabetes and health. Regular physical activity can help strengthen the heart, lungs, and bones, while also improving muscle tone, strength, and endurance. Additionally, physical activity can help control weight and body fat, lower blood pressure, and enhance the body's ability to prevent colds. It can also

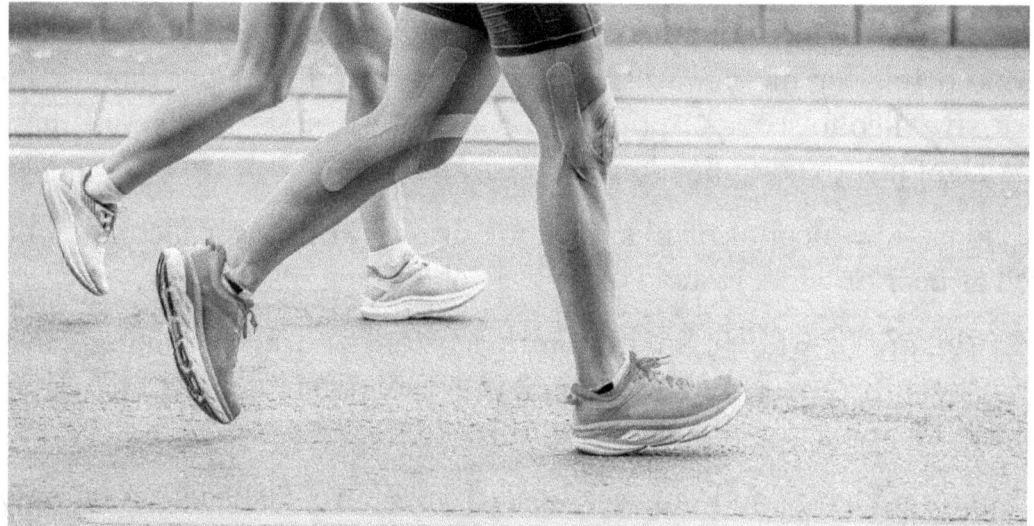

increase energy levels, reduce insulin dosage on exercise days, improve sexual function, promote better sleep, relieve stress, and boost mood.

There are various types of physical activity that can be beneficial for individuals with diabetes, including:

- Aerobic exercise: Aerobic exercise, such as brisk walking, cycling, or swimming, can help improve cardiovascular health and reduce blood sugar levels. Aim for at least 150 minutes of moderate-intensity aerobic exercise per week.

- Resistance training: Resistance training, such as weightlifting or bodyweight exercises, can help build muscle mass and increase muscle strength. This can help improve insulin sensitivity and reduce blood sugar levels. Aim for 2-3 resistance training sessions per week.

- Flexibility exercises: Flexibility exercises, such as yoga or stretching, can help improve flexibility and reduce muscle tension. This can help improve physical function and reduce the risk of injury. Aim for 2-3 flexibility exercises per week.

- High-intensity interval training (HIIT): HIIT involves short bursts of high-intensity exercise followed by brief periods of rest. HIIT can be an effective way to improve cardiovascular health and reduce blood sugar levels. Aim for 1-2 HIIT sessions per week.

Remember to consult with a healthcare provider before starting a new exercise program, especially if you have any underlying health conditions or concerns. Additionally, monitor blood sugar levels and adjust insulin dosages as needed to prevent hypoglycemia or hyperglycemia.

Physical activity is a crucial tool in managing diabetes and health. Regular physical activity can help improve cardiovascular health, reduce blood sugar levels, and enhance physical and mental well-being. By incorporating a variety of physical activities into your routine, you can improve your health and well-being.

A Few Things About Diabetes Medicine

When it comes to managing diabetes, medication can play a crucial role in helping to regulate blood sugar levels. However, it's necessary to understand

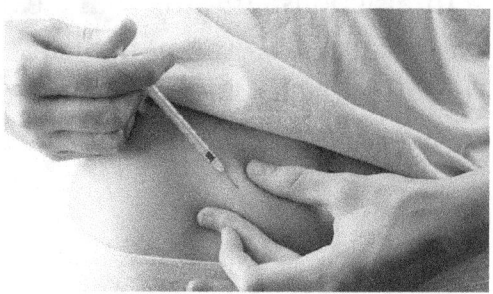

how these medications work and how they can be effectively managed. Here are some key points to consider when discussing diabetes medication with your healthcare provider:

Here are some key points to consider when discussing diabetes medication with your healthcare provider:

- Types of medication: There are several types of medication that can be used to control diabetes, including oral medications (pills) and injectable medications (insulin). Your healthcare provider will help determine which type of medication is best for you based on your individual needs.

- How they work: Oral medications work by helping your body use insulin more effectively or by producing more insulin. Insulin injections, on the other hand, provide your body with a direct source of insulin.

- Dosage and frequency: Your healthcare provider will help determine the appropriate dosage and frequency of your medication based on your individual needs. Follow their instructions carefully and not miss doses.

- Side effects: All medications can have side effects, so consider to discuss any concerns you have with your healthcare provider. They can help you manage side effects or adjust your medication regimen as needed.

- Monitoring: Keep in mind to regularly monitor your blood sugar levels to ensure that your medication is effective and to make any necessary adjustments. Your healthcare provider can help you determine the best frequency for monitoring your blood sugar levels.

- Interactions: Inform your healthcare provider of any other medications you're taking, as some medications can interact with diabetes medication. Your healthcare provider can help you avoid potential interactions and ensure that your medications are working effectively.

- Adjustments: Your healthcare provider may need to adjust your medication regimen over time based on changes in your health, lifestyle, or other factors. Follow their instructions carefully and not make any changes to your medication without their guidance.

By discussing these points with your healthcare provider, you can ensure that your diabetes medication is working effectively and safely to help manage your diabetes.

Special Tips

• Drink plenty of water. Eight (8) large glasses of water a day are recommended.

• Wear a necklace, tag, or bracelet that identifies you as a person with diabetes.

• Do physical activity with a friend.

• Wear socks and properly fitted shoes.

• Check your feet daily for blisters, redness, cuts, or open sores.

• If you don't feel well, stop the activity, check your blood glucose level, and call your doctor or primary care provider.

• Take medication as prescribed.

Living with diabetes requires you to be proactive in managing your health. Keeping track of your diabetes is essential in maintaining good health and preventing complications. Here are some tips to help you keep track of your diabetes:

- Keep a diabetes log: Keeping a log of your blood glucose levels, medication, and physical activity can help you identify patterns and make changes to manage your diabetes better. You can use a paper log or a

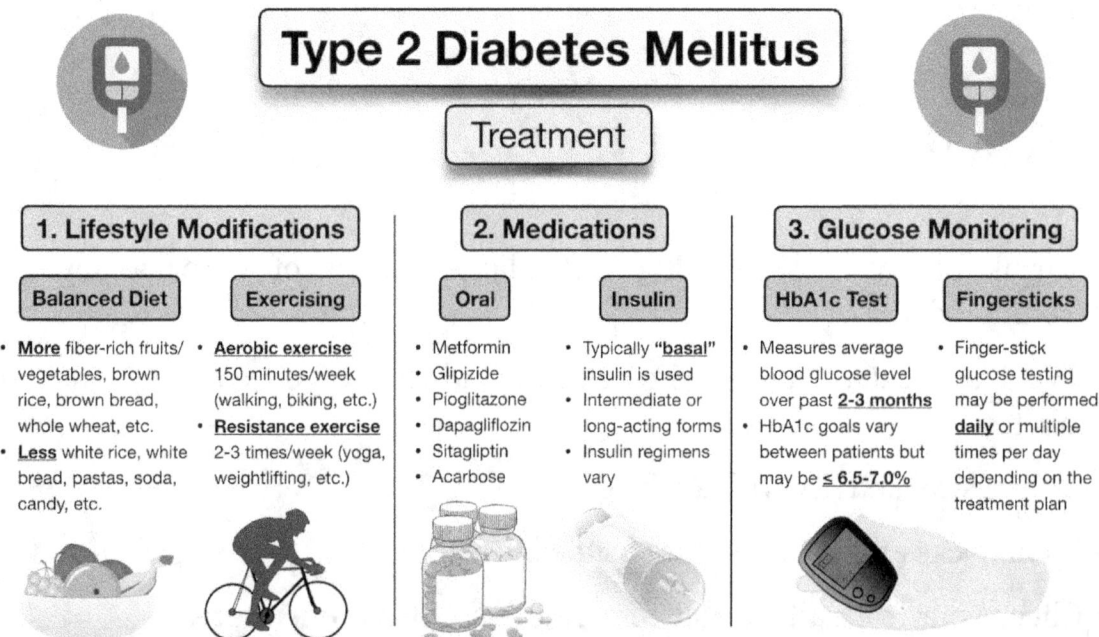

mobile app to track your data.

- Use a glucometer: A glucometer is a device that measures your blood glucose levels. It's essential to use a glucometer regularly to monitor your blood glucose levels and adjust your medication, diet, and physical activity accordingly.

- Monitor your blood pressure and cholesterol levels: High blood pressure and high cholesterol levels are common complications of diabetes. Monitoring your blood pressure and cholesterol levels regularly can help you identify any changes and take steps to manage them.

- Get regular check-ups: Regular check-ups with your doctor or primary care provider are essential in managing your diabetes. They can help you monitor your blood glucose levels, blood pressure, and cholesterol levels, and make changes to your treatment plan if necessary.

- Be aware of your medication: Keep track of your medication and dosage, and make sure you take them as prescribed. Don't skip or miss doses, and be aware of any side effects.

- Stay informed: Stay informed about diabetes and its management. Read books, articles, and online resources to learn more about diabetes and how to manage it effectively.

By keeping track of your diabetes, you can take charge of your health and prevent complications. Remember, managing diabetes requires a proactive approach, and keeping track of your health is essential in maintaining good health.

Here are some additional tips to help you keep track of your diabetes:

- Keep your diabetes log and glucometer with you at all times. This will help you track your blood glucose levels and medication dosage throughout the day.

- Set reminders on your phone or calendar to take your medication and check your blood glucose levels. This will help you stay on track and avoid missing doses or forgetting to check your levels.

- Keep a list of your medications and dosages in a visible place, such as on your fridge or in your diabetes log. This will help you remember to take your medication and avoid missed doses.

- Make a plan for managing your diabetes in case of an emergency. This could include having a spare glucometer or medication on hand, or knowing the phone number of your doctor or primary care provider.

- Consider using a diabetes management app or website to track your data and connect with other people living with diabetes. These resources can provide valuable support and help you stay motivated in managing your diabetes.

By following these tips, you can keep track of your diabetes and take charge of your health. Remember, managing diabetes requires a proactive approach, and keeping track of your health is essential in maintaining good health.

Keeping Track of Your Blood Sugar Level

BLOOD SUGAR LOG

NAME: -- MONTH: ----------------------------

DATE	TIME	LEVEL	NOTES	DATE	TIME	LEVEL	NOTES

To manage your blood sugar level effectively, it's essential to monitor it regularly. Here are some steps you can take to keep track of your blood sugar level:

- Test your blood sugar level every day: Use a glucometer to measure your blood sugar level daily, ideally before meals. This will help you understand how different foods, activities, and medications affect your blood sugar levels.

- Get a hemoglobin A1c test from your healthcare provider: This test measures your average blood sugar level over the past 2-3 months. It's an excellent way to assess your blood sugar control and make any necessary adjustments to your treatment plan. Aim to get a hemoglobin A1c test from your healthcare provider about every 3 months if you take insulin and at least every 6 months if you take oral medicine for diabetes.

- Keep a blood sugar log: Write down your blood sugar readings in a log or use a mobile app to track them. This will help you identify patterns and trends in your blood sugar levels and make it easier to manage them.

- Monitor your blood sugar levels regularly: Check your blood sugar levels regularly throughout the day, especially after meals and before bedtime. This will help you understand how different activities and foods affect your blood sugar levels and make any necessary adjustments to your treatment plan.

- Adjust your treatment plan as needed: Based on your blood sugar readings and hemoglobin A1c test results, work with your healthcare provider to adjust your treatment plan as needed. This may include changing your medication, adjusting your insulin dosage, or modifying your diet and exercise routine.

By following these steps, you can effectively keep track of your blood sugar level and manage your diabetes to live a healthy, active life.

Signs of Low Blood Sugar

Note that the signs and symptoms of low blood sugar can vary from person to person, and not everyone will experience all of them. Additionally, some people may experience different symptoms altogether. Be sure to be aware of the signs and symptoms that are specific to you, and to monitor your blood sugar levels regularly to avoid hypoglycemia.

Hypoglycemia
Common Symptoms

Shaking or tremors

Rapid heartbeat, anxiety, and panic

Hunger

Mouth tingling

Sweating

Headache and inability to concentrate

Nausea

Dizziness and weakness

If you are experiencing any of the signs or symptoms of low blood sugar, take action right away. Here are some steps you can take:

- Check your blood sugar level: Use a glucometer to check your blood sugar level. If it's below 70 mg/dL, it's considered low.

- Eat or drink something with sugar: Consuming something with sugar can help raise your blood sugar level quickly. Some examples include fruit juice, hard candy, or glucose tablets.

- Call for help: If you are unable to check your blood sugar level or if you are experiencing severe symptoms, call for emergency medical help.

- Treat with glucagon: If you are unconscious or unable to eat or drink, glucagon can be administered to help raise your blood sugar level.

Keep in mind that hypoglycemia can be a serious condition, and it's important to take it seriously. If you experience any of the signs or symptoms of low blood sugar, it's crucial to take action right away to avoid complications.

Check your blood sugar level before engaging in certain activities to ensure your safety and well-being. Low blood sugar can cause impaired judgment, reaction time, and physical abilities, which can increase the risk of injury or accident.

Here are some activities where it is important to check your blood sugar level beforehand:

- Driving a vehicle: Low blood sugar can affect your ability to drive safely, so check your blood sugar level before getting behind the wheel. If your blood sugar is low, it's best to wait until it has returned to a safe level before driving.

- Using heavy equipment: Operating heavy equipment, such as machinery or power tools, can be dangerous if your blood sugar is low. Check your blood sugar level before using any heavy equipment to ensure that you are able to operate it safely.

- Being very physically active: Engaging in strenuous physical activity can cause your blood sugar to drop rapidly. Check your blood sugar level before starting any intense physical activity, such as running, swimming, or playing sports, to make sure your levels are safe.

High Blood Sugar Symptoms To Be Aware Of

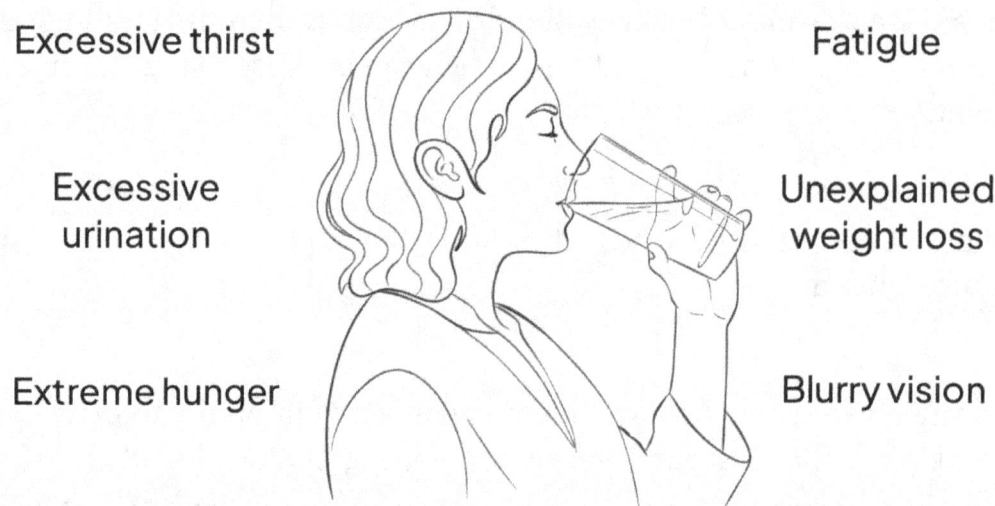

Excessive thirst

Excessive urination

Extreme hunger

Fatigue

Unexplained weight loss

Blurry vision

If you have symptoms, please reach out to your healthcare provider.

- Being active for a long time: Prolonged physical activity can also cause your blood sugar to drop. Check your blood sugar level before starting any long period of physical activity, such as a hike or a bike ride, to ensure that your levels are safe.

It's always a good idea to carry a snack or a quick source of glucose with you in case your blood sugar drops while you're engaging in these activities. This will help you quickly bring your blood sugar levels back up to a safe range.

In addition to checking your blood sugar level before these activities, it's also important to regularly monitor your blood sugar levels throughout the day to ensure that they remain within a safe range. This can help you identify any patterns or trends in your blood sugar levels and make any necessary adjustments to your diet, medication, or exercise routine.

Signs of High Blood Sugar

Signs of high blood sugar can include:

- Dry mouth: When your body has high levels of glucose in the blood, your kidneys will try to flush it out by producing more urine, which can lead to dehydration and a dry mouth.

- Thirst: As your body tries to combat the high glucose levels, it will signal your brain to drink more water, leading to feelings of thirst.

- Frequent urination: With high levels of glucose in your blood, your kidneys will work harder to filter it out, leading to more frequent trips to the bathroom.

- Feeling tired: High blood sugar levels can cause fatigue, which can make you feel weak and tired.

- Blurred vision: High blood sugar levels can cause the lens in your eye to swell, leading to blurred vision.

- Weight loss: High blood sugar levels can cause your body to burn fat for energy, leading to weight loss.

- Stomach pain, feeling sick to your stomach, or even throwing up: High blood sugar levels can cause nausea and vomiting, as well as stomach pain and discomfort.

Note that not everyone with high blood sugar will experience these symptoms, and some people may not experience any symptoms at all. However, if you do experience any of these symptoms, seek medical attention to address the underlying issue.

If you have any signs of high blood sugar, it is important to seek medical attention as soon as possible. You can start by testing your blood sugar levels at home using a glucometer, or you can visit your local health clinic or public health clinic for a blood test.

If your blood sugar levels are consistently high, your healthcare provider may diagnose you with diabetes or prediabetes. They may also recommend lifestyle changes, such as a healthy diet and regular exercise, and/or medication to help manage your blood sugar levels.

In addition to testing your blood sugar levels, your healthcare provider may also perform other tests to diagnose diabetes or prediabetes. These tests may include:

 - Fasting plasma glucose (FPG) test: This test measures your blood sugar levels after an overnight fast of at least 8 hours.

 - Oral glucose tolerance test (OGTT): This test measures your blood sugar levels after you drink a sugary drink.

 - Hemoglobin A1c (HbA1c) test: This test measures your average blood sugar levels over the past 2-3 months.

It is important to note that high blood sugar can cause serious health complications if left untreated, such as nerve damage, kidney damage, and vision loss. Therefore, it is important to seek medical attention if you experience any signs of high blood sugar.

Diabetic Eye Disease

Sure, here's a rewritten version of the article that's more concise and easier to read:

Diabetic Eye Disease: What You Need to Know

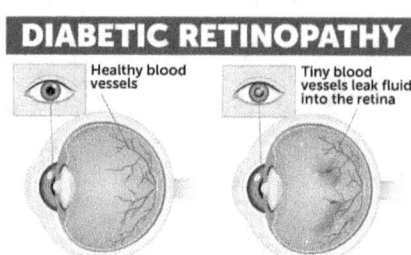

Diabetic eye disease, also known as diabetic retinopathy, is a common complication of diabetes that can cause vision loss and blindness. It occurs when high blood sugar levels damage the blood vessels in the retina, the light-sensitive tissue at the back of the eye.

Signs of Diabetic Eye Disease

The early stages of diabetic eye disease may not have any noticeable symptoms. However, as the disease progresses, you may experience:

* Blurred vision

* Double vision

* Flashes of light

* Floaters (specks or cobwebs in your vision)

* Blind spots

* Eye pain or discomfort

Be aware that these symptoms can also be caused by other eye conditions, so it's essential to have regular eye exams to determine the cause.

How to Detect Diabetic Eye Disease

The best way to detect diabetic eye disease is to have regular eye exams. Your eye doctor will perform a comprehensive eye exam to look for signs of the disease, including:

* Dilating your pupils to examine the retina and blood vessels

* Using special imaging tests, such as optical coherence tomography (OCT) or fluorescein angiography, to take pictures of the retina and blood vessels

* Checking for any signs of cataracts or other eye conditions that may be related to diabetes

If your eye doctor detects any signs of diabetic eye disease, they may recommend further testing or treatment.

Treatment for Diabetic Eye Disease

The treatment for diabetic eye disease depends on the severity of the disease. In the early stages, treatment may involve:

* Monitoring your blood sugar levels closely to prevent the disease from progressing

* Maintaining a healthy diet and exercise routine to manage your diabetes

* Taking medication to lower your blood pressure or cholesterol levels, which can help slow the progression of the disease

In more advanced cases, treatment may involve:

* Laser surgery to seal off leaking blood vessels or reduce swelling in the retina

* Injecting medication into the eye to reduce inflammation or prevent further damage

* Implanting a retinal implant to restore vision in cases of severe vision loss

Prevention is Key

The best way to prevent diabetic eye disease is to manage your diabetes carefully. This includes:

* Monitoring your blood sugar levels regularly

* Taking your medication as prescribed

* Maintaining a healthy diet and exercise routine

* Getting regular eye exams to detect any signs of the disease early

By taking these steps, you can help prevent diabetic eye disease and protect your vision.

Diabetic eye disease is a serious complication of diabetes that can cause vision loss and blindness. Early detection and treatment are key to preventing long-term damage. Regular eye exams and proper management of diabetes can help prevent or slow the progression of the disease. If you have diabetes, be sure to schedule regular eye exams and report any changes in your vision to your healthcare team or eye doctor.

Kidney Problems

Take care of your kidneys by controlling your blood sugar and blood pressure. This is important because high blood sugar and high blood pressure can damage your kidneys over time. To keep your kidneys healthy, it's necessary to manage these conditions and maintain a healthy lifestyle.

One way to check on your kidney health is to get a yearly blood test and urine test. These tests can help your healthcare provider monitor your kidney function and catch any potential problems early. If you have any

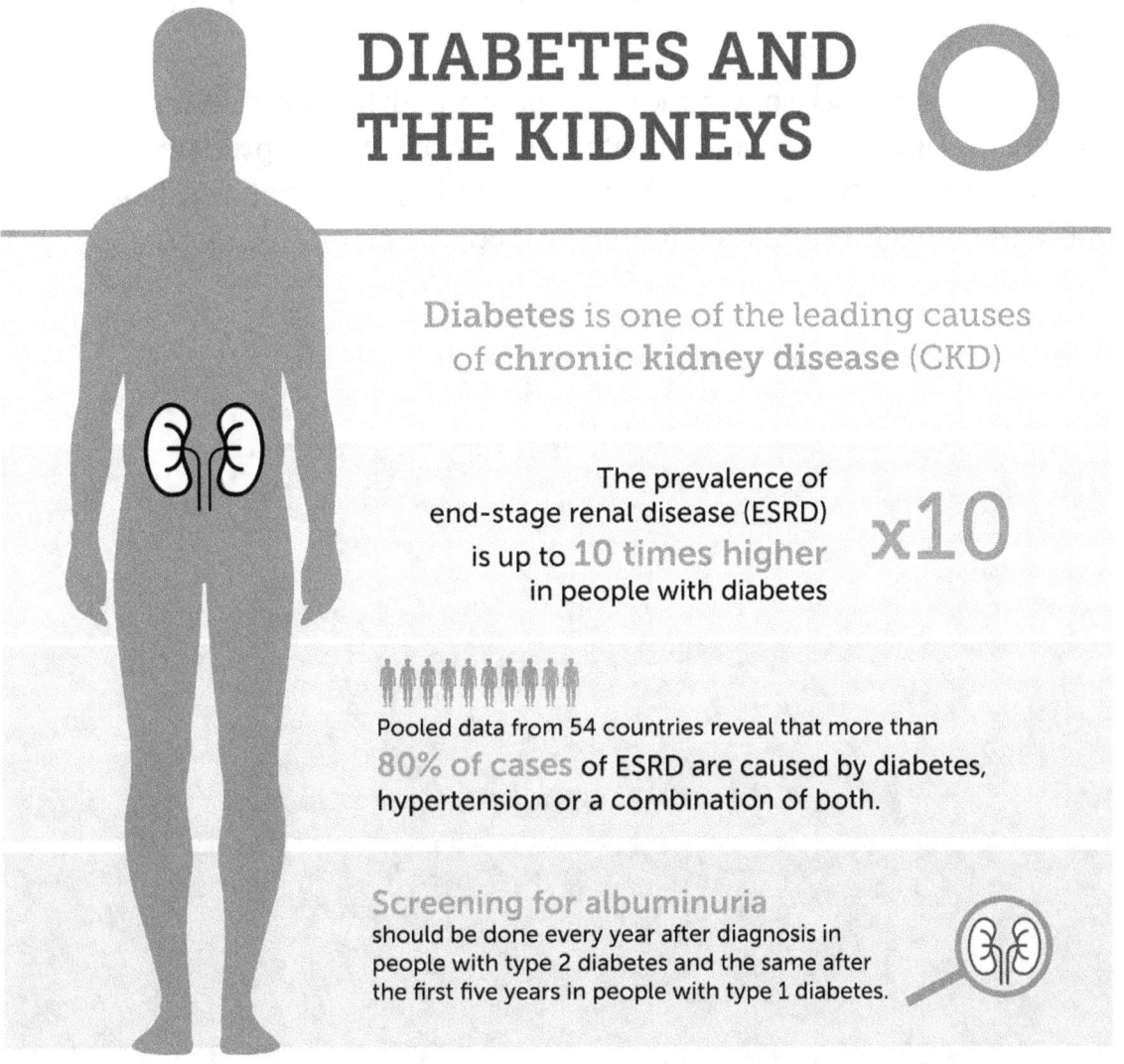

DIABETES AND THE KIDNEYS

Diabetes is one of the leading causes of **chronic kidney disease** (CKD)

The prevalence of end-stage renal disease (ESRD) is up to 10 times higher in people with diabetes

x10

Pooled data from 54 countries reveal that more than 80% of cases of ESRD are caused by diabetes, hypertension or a combination of both.

Screening for albuminuria should be done every year after diagnosis in people with type 2 diabetes and the same after the first five years in people with type 1 diabetes.

concerns or notice any changes in your urine or health, be sure to discuss them with your healthcare provider.

In addition to regular testing, it's necessary to be aware of the signs of kidney or bladder infection. These can include cloudy or bloody urine, back pain, chills, fever, and an urgent need to urinate. If you experience any of these symptoms, contact your healthcare provider right away. They can help determine the cause of the infection and provide appropriate treatment.

Remember, taking care of your kidneys is an important part of maintaining your health. By controlling your blood sugar and blood pressure, getting regular tests, and being aware of the signs of infection, you can help keep your kidneys healthy and functioning properly.

Heart and Blood Vessel Problems

When blood sugar levels are consistently high, it can damage the blood vessels and nerves, increasing the risk of heart disease and nerve damage. This can lead to a range of problems, including:

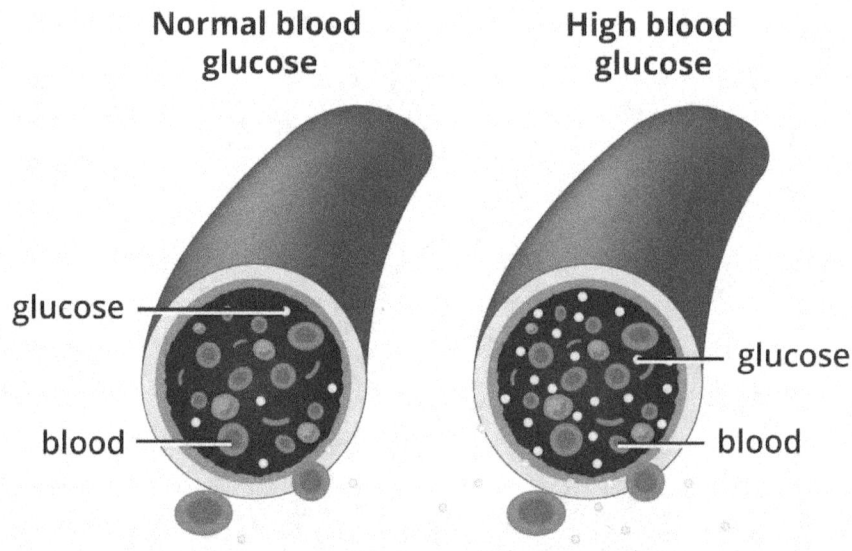

Atherosclerosis: The buildup of plaque in the arteries, which can lead to blockages and increase the risk of heart attacks and strokes.

- Heart failure: The heart becomes weakened and is unable to pump blood effectively, leading to shortness of breath, swelling, and fatigue.

- Arrhythmias: Abnormal heart rhythms, which can be dangerous and even life-threatening.

- Nerve damage: High blood sugar levels can damage the nerves, leading to numbness, tingling, and pain in the hands and feet.

- Kidney damage: The kidneys may become overworked and damaged if blood sugar levels are consistently high, leading to chronic kidney disease and potentially even kidney failure.

- Eye damage: High blood sugar levels can damage the blood vessels in the eyes, leading to vision problems and even blindness.

- Foot damage: Nerve damage and poor circulation can lead to foot ulcers and infections, which can be difficult to heal and may require amputation.

- Cognitive impairment: Diabetes has been linked to an increased risk of cognitive decline and dementia.

It's necessary for people with diabetes to work closely with their healthcare provider to manage their blood sugar levels and prevent these complications from occurring. This may involve monitoring blood sugar levels regularly, taking medication as prescribed, and making lifestyle changes such as following a healthy diet and exercising regularly.

Heart and blood vessel problems, also known as cardiovascular disease, are a major complication of diabetes. People with diabetes are at increased risk of developing heart disease, heart failure, stroke, and other cardiovascular problems. This is because high blood sugar levels can damage the blood vessels and nerves, leading to a range of complications.

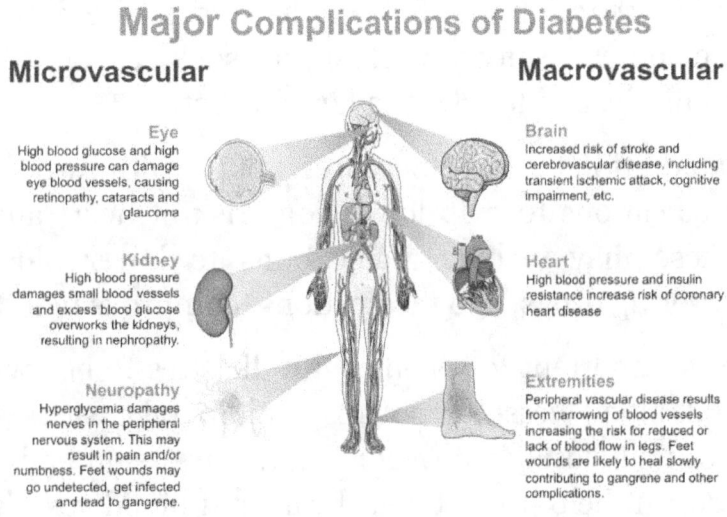

Major Complications of Diabetes

Microvascular

Eye
High blood glucose and high blood pressure can damage eye blood vessels, causing retinopathy, cataracts and glaucoma

Kidney
High blood pressure damages small blood vessels and excess blood glucose overworks the kidneys, resulting in nephropathy.

Neuropathy
Hyperglycemia damages nerves in the peripheral nervous system. This may result in pain and/or numbness. Feet wounds may go undetected, get infected and lead to gangrene.

Macrovascular

Brain
Increased risk of stroke and cerebrovascular disease, including transient ischemic attack, cognitive impairment, etc.

Heart
High blood pressure and insulin resistance increase risk of coronary heart disease

Extremities
Peripheral vascular disease results from narrowing of blood vessels increasing the risk for reduced or lack of blood flow in legs. Feet wounds are likely to heal slowly contributing to gangrene and other complications.

One of the main risks of heart and blood vessel problems is poor blood flow, also known as circulation, in the legs and feet. This can lead to pain, numbness, and tingling in the limbs, and can make it difficult to walk or stand. Poor circulation can also increase the risk of infections and ulcers, which can be difficult to heal and may require amputation.

There are several factors that can increase the risk of heart and blood vessel problems in people with diabetes. These include smoking, high blood pressure, high cholesterol, and high levels of other fats in the blood. Smoking is a major risk factor for heart disease, as it damages the blood vessels and increases the risk of blockages. High blood pressure, or hypertension, can also damage the blood vessels and increase the risk of heart disease. High cholesterol and high levels of other fats in the blood can also contribute to the development of blockages in the blood vessels.

To lower the risk of heart and blood vessel problems, it is important to work closely with your health care team. They can help you manage your blood sugar levels, blood pressure, and cholesterol levels, and can provide guidance on how often to have these levels checked. They may also recommend lifestyle changes, such as quitting smoking, exercising regularly, and following a healthy diet.

In addition to these measures, your health care team may also recommend medications to help lower your risk of heart and blood vessel problems. These may include medications to lower blood pressure, cholesterol-lowering drugs, and medications to improve blood flow to the legs and feet.

It is important for people with diabetes to be aware of their risk for heart and blood vessel problems and to take steps to reduce their risk. By working closely with your health care team and making lifestyle changes, you can help protect your heart and blood vessels and reduce your risk of complications.

Nerve Damage and Foot Problems

Diabetic Peripheral Neuropathy

Healthy Nerves and Blood Vessels

Nerves and Blood Vessels Damaged by DPN

Unmyelinated nerve fiber

Damaged unmyelinated nerve fiber

Vasa nervorum

Occluded vasa nervorum

Myelinated nerve fiber

Damaged myelinated nerve fiber

Nerve damage, also known as neuropathy, is a common complication of diabetes. It occurs when high blood sugar levels damage the nerves in the body, leading to numbness, tingling, and pain in the hands and feet. In people with diabetes, nerve damage can be particularly problematic in the feet, as it can lead to a loss of sensation and make it difficult to feel pain or discomfort.

Circulation problems, also known as peripheral artery disease, are another common complication of diabetes. This occurs when the blood vessels in the legs and feet become narrowed or blocked, reducing blood flow to the area. This can lead to a range of symptoms, including cramping, weakness, and pain in the legs and feet.

Infections that do not heal properly are another concern for people with diabetes. High blood sugar levels can weaken the immune system, making it more difficult for the body to fight off infections. This can lead to persistent infections, particularly in the feet and legs, which can be difficult to treat and may require surgical intervention.

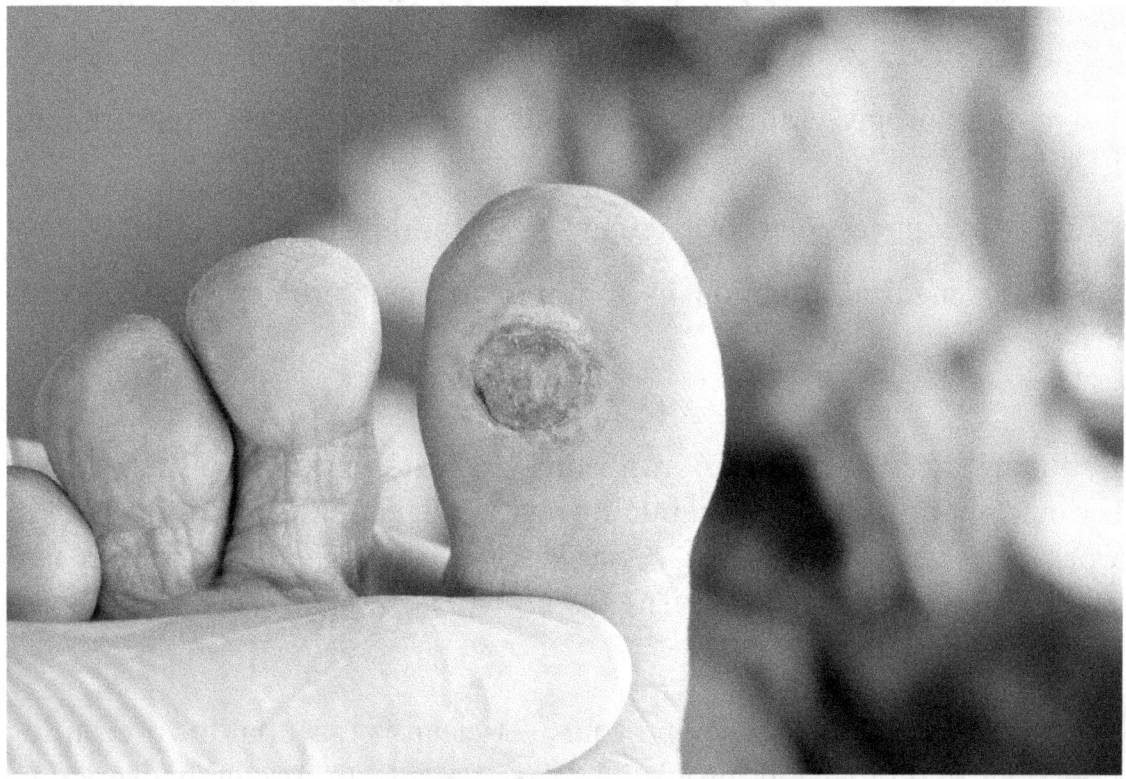

All of these factors can combine to increase the risk of serious foot problems in people with diabetes. Nerve damage can make it difficult to feel pain or discomfort, which can lead to unnoticed injuries or irritation. Circulation problems can make it difficult for wounds to heal properly, leading to prolonged healing times and an increased risk of infection. Infections that do not heal properly can spread and cause further damage, leading to serious complications such as gangrene or even amputation.

It's crucial for people with diabetes to be proactive in managing their condition and taking steps to prevent foot problems. This includes:

* Keeping blood sugar levels under control

* Monitoring and managing blood pressure and cholesterol levels

* Quitting smoking and limiting alcohol consumption

* Wearing properly fitting shoes and socks to reduce pressure and irritation

* Inspecting the feet regularly for cuts, sores, or other signs of injury

* Seeking medical attention promptly if any foot problems or concerns arise

By taking these steps, people with diabetes can help reduce their risk of serious foot problems and maintain good foot health. It's also important to work closely with a healthcare provider to manage the condition and address any foot-related concerns promptly.

 - Wash your feet daily: Keeping your feet clean is essential for preventing infections and other foot problems. Wash your feet thoroughly every day, paying special attention to the areas between your toes.

 - Check your feet daily for cracks, cuts, or blisters: Inspect your feet daily for any cuts, cracks, or blisters. If you notice any damage, seek medical attention immediately.

 - Control your blood sugar level: High blood sugar levels can damage your nerves and blood vessels, leading to foot problems. Monitor your blood sugar levels regularly and work with your healthcare provider to manage your diabetes.

- Not smoking or chewing tobacco: Smoking and chewing tobacco can damage your blood vessels and increase your risk of foot problems. Quit smoking and avoid using tobacco products.

- Not going barefooted and always wearing protective footwear: Wearing protective footwear, such as shoes or sandals, can help prevent injuries and infections. Avoid going barefooted, especially in public areas.

- Drying between your toes: Keeping your feet dry can help prevent fungal infections. Dry between your toes thoroughly after washing your feet.

By following these tips, you can help protect your feet and prevent foot problems associated with diabetes. It's also essential to work closely with your healthcare provider to manage your diabetes and monitor your foot health regularly.

Dental Disease

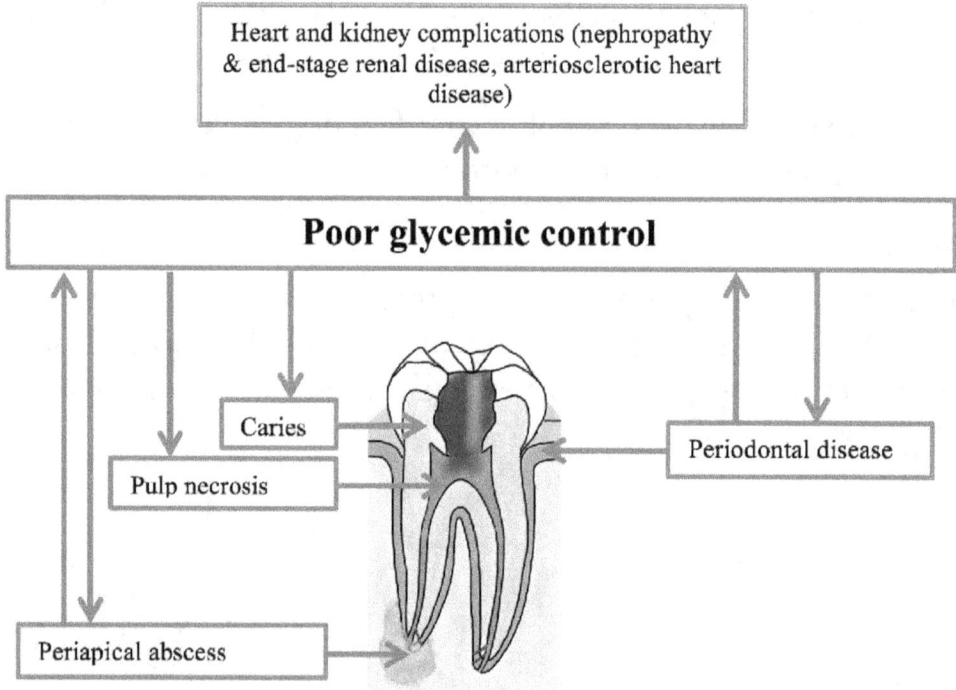

People with diabetes are at a higher risk of developing dental problems, such as tooth decay, gum disease, and dry mouth, due to their high blood sugar levels. Uncontrolled blood sugar can lead to an increase in the amount of sugar in the saliva, which can feed the bacteria in the mouth and promote the growth of harmful plaque and tartar. Additionally, high blood sugar levels can weaken the immune system, making it more difficult for the body to fight off infections and diseases in the mouth.

To protect your teeth and gums, it is important to maintain good oral hygiene habits, such as brushing your teeth at least twice a day with fluoride toothpaste and cleaning between your teeth once a day with floss or an interdental cleaner. It is also recommended to visit your dentist for regular check-ups and cleanings every six months. Your dentist can help you identify any early signs of dental problems and provide you with personalized recommendations for maintaining good oral health.

In addition to good oral hygiene habits, controlling your blood sugar levels is also crucial for maintaining healthy teeth and gums. This can be achieved through a combination of a healthy diet, regular exercise, and medication, if necessary. By working closely with your healthcare provider and practicing good oral hygiene, you can help prevent dental problems associated with diabetes and maintain a healthy, beautiful smile.

Vaccinations

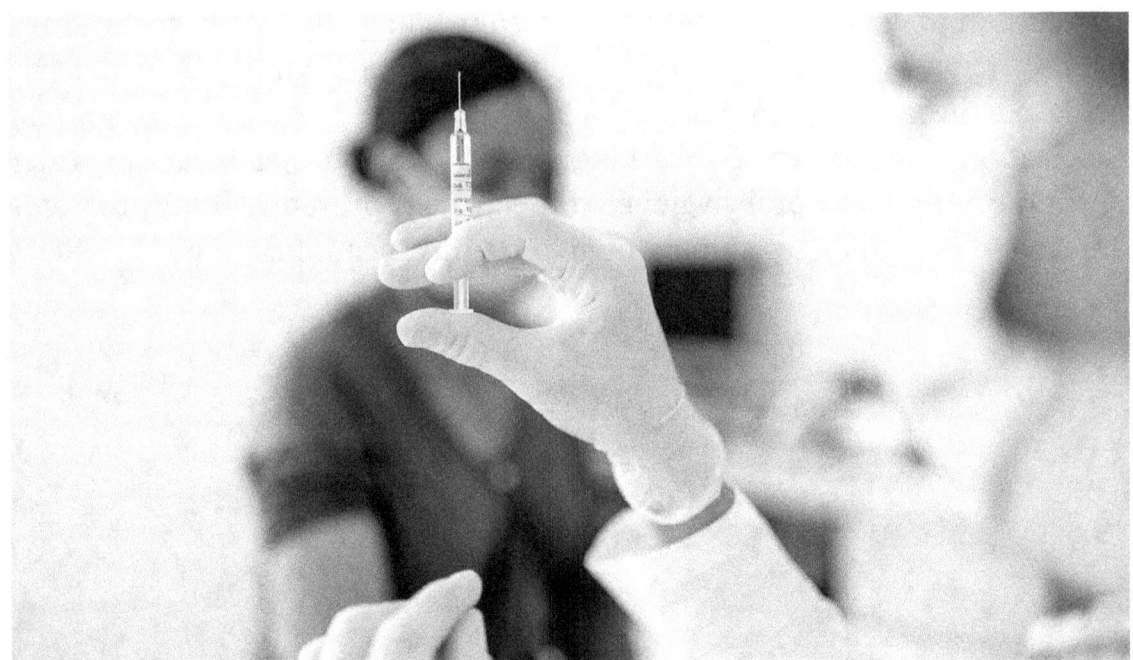

"Did you know that getting a yearly flu shot can help prevent serious complications from the flu, such as pneumonia, bronchitis, and sinus and ear infections? And if you have diabetes, it's especially important to get vaccinated, as you're at a higher risk for complications from the flu. Talk to your healthcare team or doctor about getting vaccinated today!

This tweet emphasizes the importance of getting a flu shot for people with diabetes, as they are at a higher risk for complications from the flu. It also includes a call to action, encouraging readers to talk to their healthcare team or doctor about getting vaccinated. The hashtags #DiabetesAwareness and #FluPrevention help to reach a wider audience and raise awareness about the importance of vaccination for people with diabetes.

There are several other ways that people with diabetes can protect themselves from the flu:

- Get vaccinated: The flu vaccine is the most effective way to prevent the flu. People with diabetes should get vaccinated every year, ideally by the end of October.

- Practice good hygiene: Wash your hands frequently with soap and water, especially after coughing or sneezing. Avoid touching your eyes, nose, and mouth as these are common entry points for germs.

- Avoid close contact with people who are sick: Try to keep a distance of at least 6 feet from people who are sick with the flu.

- Stay home when sick: If you're sick with the flu, stay home from work or school to avoid spreading the flu to others.

- Keep your blood sugar levels under control: People with diabetes should make sure to keep their blood sugar levels under control to help prevent complications from the flu.

- Get enough sleep: Lack of sleep can weaken the immune system, making it easier to get sick. Aim for 7-8 hours of sleep per night.

- Stay hydrated: Drink plenty of water and clear liquids to help keep your body hydrated and your immune system functioning properly.

- Manage stress: High levels of stress can weaken the immune system, making it easier to get sick. Try to manage stress through relaxation techniques like meditation or deep breathing.

People with diabetes may face specific complications from the flu, including:

- Pneumonia: The flu can lead to pneumonia, a serious infection that can cause breathing problems and hospitalization. People with diabetes are at a higher risk for developing pneumonia from the flu.

- Bronchitis: The flu can also lead to bronchitis, an infection of the airways that can cause coughing, wheezing, and difficulty breathing.

- Sinus and ear infections: The flu can lead to sinus and ear infections, which can cause pain, congestion, and hearing loss.

- Worsening of diabetes control: The flu can make it harder to control blood sugar levels, which can lead to serious complications like hypoglycemia (low blood sugar) or hyperglycemia (high blood sugar).

- Increased risk of cardiovascular problems: The flu can increase the risk of cardiovascular problems, such as heart attacks and strokes, in people with diabetes.

There are several flu vaccines that are recommended for people with diabetes, including:

- The trivalent flu vaccine (TIV): This vaccine protects against three strains of the flu virus and is recommended for people with diabetes who are under the age of 6 -

- The quadrivalent flu vaccine (QIV): This vaccine protects against four strains of the flu virus and is recommended for people with diabetes who are over the age of 6 -

- The high-dose flu vaccine: This vaccine contains four times the amount of antigen as the standard-dose vaccine and is recommended for people with diabetes who are over the age of 6 -

- The adjuvanted flu vaccine: This vaccine contains an adjuvant, which helps to stimulate the immune system and is recommended for people with diabetes who are over the age of 6 -

Note that the specific recommendations for flu vaccines may vary depending on the individual's age, health status, and other factors, so it's best to consult with a healthcare provider to determine the most appropriate vaccine.

What are the common side effects of the high-dose flu vaccine for people with diabetes? More information about the adjuvanted flu vaccine and how it works. Are there any additional precautions people with diabetes should take during flu season?

The high-dose flu vaccine, also known as the influenza vaccine high-dose (HD), is a type of flu vaccine that contains four times the amount of antigen as the standard-dose flu vaccine. It is recommended for people aged 65 and older, including those with diabetes, as it has been shown to be more effective in preventing flu in this age group.

Common side effects of the high-dose flu vaccine for people with diabetes are similar to those of the standard-dose flu vaccine and may include:

* Pain, redness, or swelling at the injection site

* Fatigue

* Headache

* Muscle aches

* Fever

* Chills

* Nausea

These side effects are generally mild and temporary, and they go away on their own within a few days.

The adjuvanted flu vaccine, also known as the MF59-adjuvanted flu vaccine, is a type of flu vaccine that contains an adjuvant called MF5 - An adjuvant is a substance that helps to stimulate the immune system and increase the body's response to the vaccine. The MF59 adjuvant is made from a mixture of water, oil, and a small amount of a chemical called squalene. It is added to the flu vaccine to help the body produce a stronger immune response and provide better protection against the flu.

The adjuvanted flu vaccine is recommended for people aged 65 and older, including those with diabetes, as it has been shown to be more effective in preventing flu in this age group.

In addition to getting vaccinated, there are several additional precautions that people with diabetes can take during flu season to protect themselves from the flu:

 - Practice good hygiene: Wash your hands frequently with soap and water, especially after coughing or sneezing. Avoid touching your eyes, nose, and mouth as these are common entry points for germs.

 - Avoid close contact with people who are sick: Try to keep a distance of at least 6 feet from people who are sick with the flu.

 - Stay home when sick: If you're sick with the flu, stay home from work or school to avoid spreading the flu to others.

- Keep your blood sugar levels under control: People with diabetes should make sure to keep their blood sugar levels under control to help prevent complications from the flu.

- Get enough sleep: Lack of sleep can weaken the immune system, making it easier to get sick. Aim for 7-8 hours of sleep per night.

- Stay hydrated: Drink plenty of water and clear liquids to help keep your body hydrated and your immune system functioning properly.

- Manage stress: High levels of stress can weaken the immune system, making it easier to get sick. Try to manage stress through relaxation techniques like meditation or deep breathing.

- Consider taking antiviral medication: If you do get sick with the flu, consider taking antiviral medication such as oseltamivir (Tamiflu) or zanamivir (Relenza) to help reduce the severity and duration of your symptoms. These medications work best when started within 48 hours of symptoms first appearing.

These precautions are especially important for people with diabetes, as they are at a higher risk for complications from the flu. By taking these steps, you can help protect yourself and others from the flu during flu season.

Questions and Answers

What are some common risk factors for developing diabetes? Can you explain how insulin works in the body? Are there any natural remedies or alternative treatments for diabetes?

Common risk factors for developing diabetes include:

* Genetics: Having a family history of diabetes can increase a person's risk of developing the disease.

* Obesity: Being overweight or obese can increase a person's risk of developing type 2 diabetes, as excess body fat can increase resistance to insulin.

* Physical inactivity: A sedentary lifestyle can increase a person's risk of developing type 2 diabetes, as regular physical activity helps to improve insulin sensitivity.

* Age: The risk of developing type 2 diabetes increases with age, especially after the age of 4 -

* Ethnicity: Certain ethnic groups, such as African Americans, Hispanics/Latinos, and Native Americans, have a higher risk of developing type 2 diabetes.

* History of gestational diabetes: Women who have had gestational diabetes during pregnancy are at increased risk of developing type 2 diabetes later in life.

* Polycystic ovary syndrome (PCOS): Women with PCOS are at higher risk of developing insulin resistance and type 2 diabetes.

* Sleep apnea: People with sleep apnea are at higher risk of developing type 2 diabetes, as sleep apnea can disrupt normal sleep patterns and increase inflammation in the body.

* Certain medications: Some medications, such as corticosteroids and certain psychiatric medications, can increase a person's risk of developing type 2 diabetes.

Insulin is a hormone produced by the pancreas that helps to regulate blood sugar levels in the body. Insulin works by binding to insulin receptors on the surface of cells, which triggers a cascade of signaling pathways that ultimately lead to the uptake of glucose by the cells. Insulin also helps to regulate the storage of glucose in the liver and muscles, and it plays a role in the metabolism of fat and protein.

There are several natural remedies and alternative treatments for diabetes that have been studied, including:

* Cinnamon: Cinnamon has been shown to improve insulin sensitivity and reduce blood sugar levels in people with type 2 diabetes.

* Berberine: Berberine is a compound found in the Berberis genus of plants that has been shown to improve insulin sensitivity and reduce blood sugar levels in people with type 2 diabetes.

* Bitter melon: Bitter melon is a fruit that has been used in traditional medicine for centuries to treat diabetes. It has been shown to improve insulin sensitivity and reduce blood sugar levels in people with type 2 diabetes.

* Gymnema sylvestre: Gymnema sylvestre is a plant that has been used in traditional medicine for centuries to treat diabetes. It has been shown to

improve insulin sensitivity and reduce blood sugar levels in people with type 2 diabetes.

* Turmeric: Turmeric contains a compound called curcumin that has been shown to have anti-inflammatory and antioxidant properties, which may help to reduce the risk of complications associated with diabetes.

* alpha-lipoic acid: Alpha-lipoic acid is an antioxidant that has been shown to improve insulin sensitivity and reduce nerve damage in people with diabetes.

Note that while these natural remedies and alternative treatments may be helpful in managing diabetes, they should not be used as a substitute for conventional treatment. It's crucial to work with a healthcare provider to develop a comprehensive treatment plan that includes lifestyle modifications, medication, and other therapies as needed.

Can you provide more information on how cinnamon improves insulin sensitivity? What are some lifestyle modifications that can help manage diabetes? Are there any potential side effects or risks associated with using natural remedies for diabetes?

Cinnamon has been shown to improve insulin sensitivity in several ways:

  - Increasing glucose uptake: Cinnamon has been shown to increase the uptake of glucose by the cells, which can help to lower blood sugar levels.

  - Improving insulin signaling: Cinnamon has been shown to improve the signaling of insulin receptors, which can help to improve the body's ability to use insulin effectively.

- Reducing inflammation: Cinnamon has anti-inflammatory properties, which can help to reduce inflammation in the body, which is a common complication of diabetes.

- Improving blood vessel function: Cinnamon has been shown to improve blood vessel function, which can help to reduce the risk of complications associated with diabetes, such as heart disease and stroke.

Lifestyle modifications that can help manage diabetes include:

- Healthy diet: Eating a healthy, balanced diet that is low in sugar, salt, and saturated fats can help to manage diabetes.

- Regular exercise: Regular physical activity can help to improve insulin sensitivity and reduce blood sugar levels.

- Maintaining a healthy weight: Maintaining a healthy weight can help to reduce the risk of complications associated with diabetes.

- Stress management: Stress can raise blood sugar levels and worsen diabetes symptoms. Engaging in stress-reducing activities, such as yoga, meditation, or deep breathing, can help to manage stress.

- Getting enough sleep: Getting enough sleep is important for health and can help to manage diabetes symptoms.

There are some potential side effects and risks associated with using natural remedies for diabetes, including:

- Interaction with medications: Some natural remedies, such as cinnamon, can interact with medications and affect blood sugar levels. It's imperative to talk to a healthcare provider before taking any natural remedies.

- Allergic reactions: Some people may be allergic to certain natural remedies, such as cinnamon, and experience an allergic reaction.

- Lowering blood sugar too much: Some natural remedies, such as cinnamon, can lower blood sugar levels too much, which can be dangerous. Monitor blood sugar levels closely when using natural remedies.

- Quality and purity: The quality and purity of natural remedies can vary, and some may contain harmful ingredients. Choose a reputable brand and follow the recommended dosage.

Natural remedies should not be used as a substitute for conventional treatment. It's necessary to work with a healthcare provider to develop a comprehensive treatment plan that includes lifestyle modifications, medication, and other therapies as needed.

What are some other natural remedies that have been shown to be effective for managing diabetes? Can you provide more information on how stress management can help with managing diabetes? Are there any specific types of exercise that are particularly beneficial for managing diabetes?

Here are some other natural remedies that have been shown to be effective for managing diabetes:

- Berberine: Berberine is a compound found in the Berberis genus of plants that has been shown to improve insulin sensitivity and reduce blood sugar levels.

- Bitter melon: Bitter melon, also known as Momordica charantia, is a fruit that has been used in traditional medicine for centuries to treat diabetes. It has been shown to improve insulin sensitivity and reduce blood sugar levels.

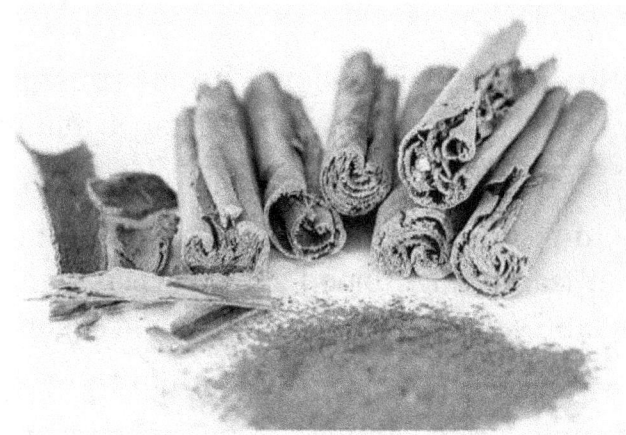

- Gymnema sylvestre: Gymnema sylvestre is a plant that has been used in traditional medicine for centuries to treat diabetes. It has been shown to improve insulin sensitivity and reduce blood sugar levels.

- Turmeric: Turmeric contains a compound called curcumin that has anti-inflammatory and antioxidant properties, which can help to reduce inflammation and improve insulin sensitivity.

- Cinnamon: Cinnamon has been shown to improve insulin sensitivity and reduce blood sugar levels.

- alpha-lipoic acid: Alpha-lipoic acid is an antioxidant that has been shown to improve insulin sensitivity and reduce nerve damage in people with diabetes.

- Magnesium: Magnesium is a mineral that can help to improve insulin sensitivity and reduce blood pressure.

- Chromium: Chromium is a mineral that can help to improve insulin sensitivity and reduce blood sugar levels.

- Vanadium: Vanadium is a mineral that can help to improve insulin sensitivity and reduce blood sugar levels.

Stress management can help with managing diabetes in several ways:

- Reduces inflammation: Chronic stress can lead to chronic inflammation, which can worsen insulin resistance and increase the risk of complications associated with diabetes.

- Improves insulin sensitivity: Stress can impair insulin sensitivity, which can lead to high blood sugar levels. Managing stress can help to improve insulin sensitivity and reduce blood sugar levels.

- Improves blood sugar control: Stress can raise blood sugar levels, and chronic stress can lead to poor blood sugar control. Managing stress can help to improve blood sugar control and reduce the risk of complications associated with diabetes.

- Reduces cortisol levels: Cortisol is a hormone produced by the adrenal glands in response to stress. High cortisol levels can lead to insulin resistance and weight gain, which can worsen diabetes symptoms. Managing stress can help to reduce cortisol levels and improve insulin sensitivity.

There are several types of exercise that are particularly beneficial for managing diabetes, including:

- Aerobic exercise: Aerobic exercise, such as brisk walking, cycling, or swimming, can help to improve insulin sensitivity and reduce blood sugar levels.

- Resistance training: Resistance training, such as weightlifting or bodyweight exercises, can help to build muscle mass and improve insulin sensitivity.

- Yoga: Yoga combines physical movement with deep breathing and relaxation techniques, which can help to reduce stress and improve insulin sensitivity.

- High-intensity interval training (HIIT): HIIT involves short bursts of high-intensity exercise followed by periods of rest. This type of exercise has been shown to improve insulin sensitivity and reduce blood sugar levels.

- Tai chi: Tai chi is a form of martial arts that involves slow, flowing movements that can help to improve balance, flexibility, and insulin sensitivity.

Everyone is different, and the best exercise plan for managing diabetes will depend on individual factors such as fitness level, health status, and lifestyle. Consult with a healthcare provider or a certified fitness professional to develop a safe and effective exercise plan.

Can you provide more information on the benefits of resistance training for managing diabetes? What are some other natural remedies that can help reduce inflammation in the body? How can I determine the right intensity and duration for aerobic exercise to manage diabetes?

Resistance training, also known as strength training, can have numerous benefits for individuals with diabetes. Here are some of the ways it can help:

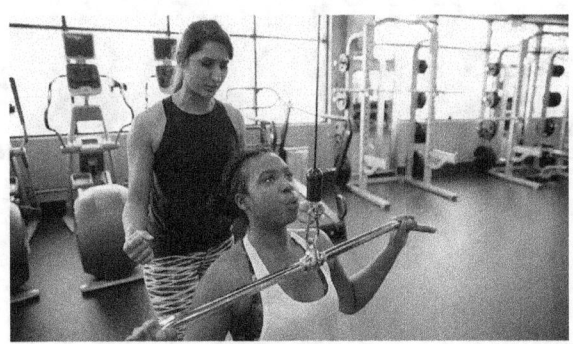

- Improved insulin sensitivity: Resistance training can help improve insulin sensitivity, which means that the body's cells become better at using insulin to uptake glucose from the bloodstream. This can help regulate blood sugar levels and improve glucose metabolism.

- Increased muscle mass: Resistance training can help build muscle mass, which can increase the body's metabolic rate and help burn more calories, including glucose. This can help regulate blood sugar levels and improve glucose metabolism.

- Improved blood lipid profiles: Resistance training can help improve blood lipid profiles by increasing levels of high-density lipoprotein (HDL) cholesterol and reducing levels of low-density lipoprotein (LDL) cholesterol. This can help reduce the risk of cardiovascular disease, which is a common complication of diabetes.

- Reduced inflammation: Resistance training can help reduce inflammation in the body, which is a key factor in the development of insulin resistance and other complications of diabetes.

- Improved mental health: Resistance training can help improve mental health by reducing stress and anxiety levels, which can be beneficial for individuals with diabetes who may experience emotional distress related to their condition.

Other natural remedies that can help reduce inflammation in the body include:

- Omega-3 fatty acids: These anti-inflammatory fatty acids can be found in fatty fish, flaxseed, and other foods.

- Turmeric: The active compound curcumin in turmeric has potent anti-inflammatory properties.

- Ginger: Ginger has anti-inflammatory properties and can help reduce inflammation in the body.

- Berries: Berries such as blueberries, raspberries, and strawberries are rich in antioxidants and can help reduce inflammation.

- Green tea: Green tea contains polyphenols, which can help reduce inflammation and improve health.

To determine the right intensity and duration for aerobic exercise to manage diabetes, consult with a healthcare provider or a certified fitness professional. They can help you develop a safe and effective exercise plan based on your individual needs and health status.

In general, aerobic exercise for diabetes management should be moderate-intensity and duration. Moderate-intensity exercise is typically defined as exercise that raises your heart rate and causes you to break a sweat, but still allows you to carry on a conversation. Examples of moderate-intensity aerobic exercise include brisk walking, cycling, swimming, and dancing.

The duration of aerobic exercise for diabetes management can vary depending on the individual, but aim for at least 150 minutes of moderate-intensity aerobic exercise per week. This can be broken up into shorter sessions throughout the week, such as 30 minutes per day, five days per week.

Remember to always monitor your blood sugar levels before, during, and after exercise, and to carry a source of fast-acting carbohydrates with you in case of hypoglycemia. It's also important to listen to your body and adjust your exercise plan as needed based on how you feel.

What are some other types of moderate-intensity aerobic exercises that can be beneficial for managing diabetes? Can you provide more information on the potential risks or precautions associated with resistance training for individuals with diabetes? Are there any specific guidelines for incorporating resistance training into a diabetes management plan?

Other types of moderate-intensity aerobic exercises that can be beneficial for managing diabetes include:

- Brisk walking: Walking quickly at a pace of about 3-4 miles per hour can help improve cardiovascular health and regulate blood sugar levels.

- Swimming: Swimming is a low-impact exercise that can help improve cardiovascular health and strengthen muscles without putting excessive strain on the joints.

- Cycling: Cycling can be an effective way to improve cardiovascular health and regulate blood sugar levels, especially if done at a moderate to high intensity.

- Dancing: Dancing can be a fun and effective way to improve cardiovascular health and regulate blood sugar levels, especially if done at a moderate to high intensity.

- Aerobics: Participating in group aerobics classes or following along with aerobics videos at home can be a great way to get a moderate-intensity workout and improve cardiovascular health.

Potential risks or precautions associated with resistance training for individuals with diabetes include:

- Hypoglycemia: Resistance training can cause blood sugar levels to drop, so monitor blood sugar levels before, during, and after exercise.

- Injury: Resistance training can be strenuous and may lead to injury if proper form and technique are not used. Work with a qualified fitness professional to learn proper form and technique.

- Muscle strain: Resistance training can cause muscle strain, especially if proper warm-up and cool-down exercises are not performed.

- Overexertion: Resistance training can be strenuous and may lead to overexertion if proper intensity and duration are not monitored.

Guidelines for incorporating resistance training into a diabetes management plan include:

- Consult with a healthcare provider: Before starting any new exercise program, make sure to consult with a healthcare provider to ensure that it's safe and appropriate for your individual needs.

- Start slowly: Begin with low-intensity resistance training exercises and gradually increase the intensity and duration over time.

- Monitor blood sugar levels: Monitor blood sugar levels before, during, and after exercise to ensure that they remain within a safe range.

- Use proper form and technique: Work with a qualified fitness professional to learn proper form and technique to avoid injury.

- Incorporate a variety of exercises: Incorporate a variety of exercises into your resistance training program to ensure that all major muscle groups are being targeted.

- Gradually increase intensity and duration: Gradually increase the intensity and duration of your resistance training program over time to avoid overexertion and ensure that you're making progress.

- Stretch and cool down: Always stretch and cool down after resistance training exercises to help prevent muscle strain and improve flexibility.

Be sure to remember that everyone's health and fitness needs are different, so to consult with a healthcare provider or a certified fitness professional to develop a personalized exercise plan that's safe and effective for managing diabetes.

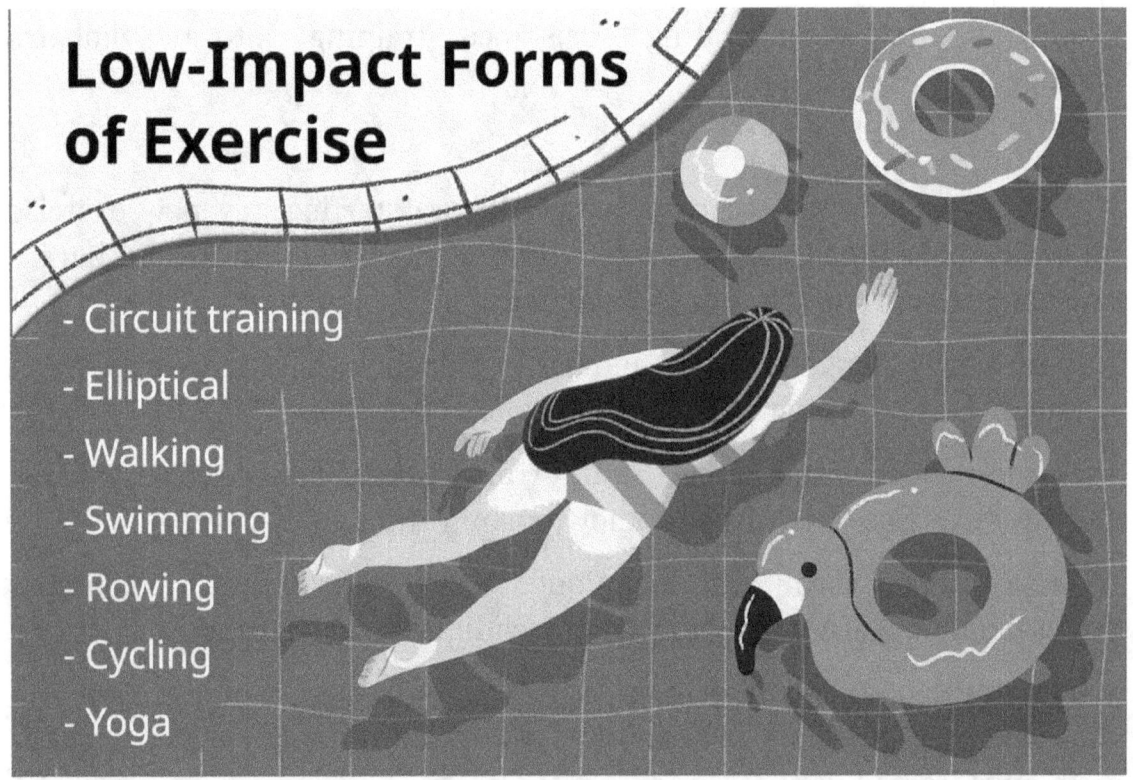

What are some other low-impact exercises that can be beneficial for managing diabetes? Can you provide more information on the potential risks or precautions associated with aerobic exercises for individuals with diabetes? Are there any specific guidelines for incorporating aerobic exercises into a diabetes management plan?

Other low-impact exercises that can be beneficial for managing diabetes include:

- Yoga: Yoga can help improve flexibility, balance, and strength, and can also help reduce stress and improve well-being.

- Pilates: Pilates is a form of exercise that focuses on core strength, flexibility, and body control. It can help improve posture, balance, and muscle tone.

- Swimming: Swimming is a low-impact exercise that can help improve cardiovascular health and strengthen muscles without putting excessive strain on the joints.

- Cycling: Cycling is a low-impact exercise that can help improve cardiovascular health and strengthen muscles in the legs.

- Tai chi: Tai chi is a form of martial arts that involves slow, flowing movements that can help improve balance, flexibility, and strength.

Potential risks or precautions associated with aerobic exercises for individuals with diabetes include:

- Hypoglycemia: Aerobic exercise can cause blood sugar levels to drop, so be sure to monitor blood sugar levels before, during, and after exercise.

- Injury: Aerobic exercise can be strenuous and may lead to injury if proper form and technique are not used. Work with a qualified fitness professional to learn proper form and technique.

- Overexertion: Aerobic exercise can be strenuous and may lead to overexertion if proper intensity and duration are not monitored.

- Dehydration: Aerobic exercise can cause dehydration, so make sure to drink plenty of water before, during, and after exercise.

Guidelines for incorporating aerobic exercises into a diabetes management plan include:

- Consult with a healthcare provider: Before starting any new exercise program, consult with a healthcare provider to ensure that it's safe and appropriate for your individual needs.

- Start slowly: Begin with low-intensity aerobic exercises and gradually increase the intensity and duration over time.

- Monitor blood sugar levels: Monitor blood sugar levels before, during, and after exercise to ensure that they remain within a safe range.

- Use proper form and technique: Work with a qualified fitness professional to learn proper form and technique to avoid injury.

- Incorporate a variety of exercises: Incorporate a variety of aerobic exercises into your program to ensure that all major muscle groups are being targeted.

- Gradually increase intensity and duration: Gradually increase the intensity and duration of your aerobic exercise program over time to avoid overexertion and ensure that you're making progress.

- Stretch and cool down: Always stretch and cool down after aerobic exercise to help prevent muscle strain and improve flexibility.

Remember that everyone's health and fitness needs are different, so with a healthcare provider or a certified fitness professional to develop a personalized exercise plan that's safe and effective for managing diabetes.

Are there any specific guidelines for incorporating strength training exercises into a diabetes management plan?

Yes, there are specific guidelines for incorporating strength training exercises into a diabetes management plan. The American Diabetes Association (ADA) recommends that individuals with diabetes incorporate strength training exercises into their fitness routine to help manage their blood sugar levels and health.

Exercise Type	Description	Blood Glucose Effects
Aerobic	Lower intensity, longer duration	Expect a drop in glucose levels
Anaerobic	Higher intensity, shorter duration	Expect spikes in glucose levels
Mixed	Combination of aerobic and anaerobic activity	Expect glucose levels to fluctuate, can drop or spike

Here are some guidelines for incorporating strength training exercises into a diabetes management plan:

  - Consult with a healthcare provider: Before starting any new exercise program, consult with a healthcare provider to ensure that it's safe and appropriate for your individual needs.

  - Start slowly: Begin with low-intensity strength training exercises and gradually increase the intensity and duration over time.

  - Focus on compound exercises: Compound exercises, such as squats, deadlifts, and bench press, are effective for building muscle mass and improving strength.

- Incorporate exercises for all major muscle groups: Incorporate exercises that target all major muscle groups, including the legs, hips, back, shoulders, chest, and arms.

- Use proper form and technique: Work with a qualified fitness professional to learn proper form and technique to avoid injury and ensure that you're targeting the correct muscles.

- Incorporate progressive overload: Gradually increase the weight or resistance used in your strength training exercises over time to continue challenging your muscles and promoting strength gains.

- Aim for 2-3 strength training sessions per week: Aim for 2-3 strength training sessions per week, with at least one day of rest in between.

- Monitor blood sugar levels: Monitor your blood sugar levels before, during, and after strength training exercises to ensure that they remain within a safe range.

- Consider incorporating resistance band exercises: Resistance band exercises can be a great option for individuals with diabetes who may have mobility or strength limitations.

- Be consistent: Consistency is key when it comes to incorporating strength training exercises into a diabetes management plan. Aim to make strength training a regular part of your fitness routine.

Remember, work with a qualified fitness professional to develop a personalized strength training program that's safe and effective for managing diabetes. They can help you develop a program that takes into account your individual needs and health status.

How can I stay motivated and engaged in my diabetes self-care routine over time?

Staying motivated and engaged in your diabetes self-care routine can be challenging, but there are several strategies that can help. Here are some tips:

- Set clear and achievable goals: Setting specific, measurable, and attainable goals can help you stay motivated and focused. Break down your goals into smaller, manageable steps, and track your progress over time.

- Make it a habit: Incorporate your diabetes self-care routine into your daily routine, so it becomes a habit. Try to perform your routine at the same time every day, so it becomes second nature.

MOTIVATION

- Watch a motivational TedTalk or other video
- Listen to a motivational podcast
- Journal
- Use a mental health app
- Plan out your day/week
- Make a list of short term and long term goals with ways to achieve them
- Make a highs/lows list, (or just a highs list if you notice that you always include too many lows)
- Create a vision board
- Fill in your calendar
- Write positive affirmations and things you love about yourself
- Make a healthy habit tracking log
- Try on your favorite outfits that make you confident
- Create a bucket list
- Read inspirational quotes
- Write a letter to your future self
- Watch a how-to video on something you've wanted to try

- Find support: Connect with others who have diabetes, either in person or online. Sharing experiences and tips can help you stay motivated and inspired. Join a diabetes support group, attend diabetes conferences, or participate in online forums.

- Celebrate milestones: Celebrate your successes, no matter how small. Recognize and reward yourself for reaching your goals, like a week of healthy eating or a month of consistent exercise.

- Get creative: Find ways to make your self-care routine more enjoyable. Listen to music, watch a movie, or read a book while exercising, or try new recipes that are healthy and delicious.

- Take breaks: It's necessary to take breaks and rest when you need to. Don't be too hard on yourself if you miss a day or two. Get back on track as soon as you can, and don't let a minor setback discourage you.

- Stay informed: Stay up-to-date with the latest diabetes research, treatments, and management strategies. Attend diabetes education workshops, read diabetes publications, or follow diabetes experts on social media.

- Make it a family affair: Involve your family and friends in your diabetes self-care routine. Share your goals, progress, and successes with them, and ask for their support and encouragement.

- Be kind to yourself: Remember that managing diabetes is a journey, and it's okay to have ups and downs. Don't be too hard on yourself if you make mistakes or have setbacks. Instead, focus on what you can do to improve your self-care routine moving forward.

- Seek professional help: If you're struggling to stay motivated or engaged in your diabetes self-care routine, consider seeking help from a mental health professional. They can help you develop coping strategies and provide support and guidance when needed.

Remember, managing diabetes requires a long-term commitment to healthy lifestyle habits and self-care. By staying motivated and engaged, you can improve your health and well-being, and enjoy a better quality of life.

How can I involve my family and friends in my diabetes self-care routine?

Involving your family and friends in your diabetes self-care routine can be a great way to build a support system and make managing your diabetes easier and more enjoyable. Here are some ways to involve your loved ones:

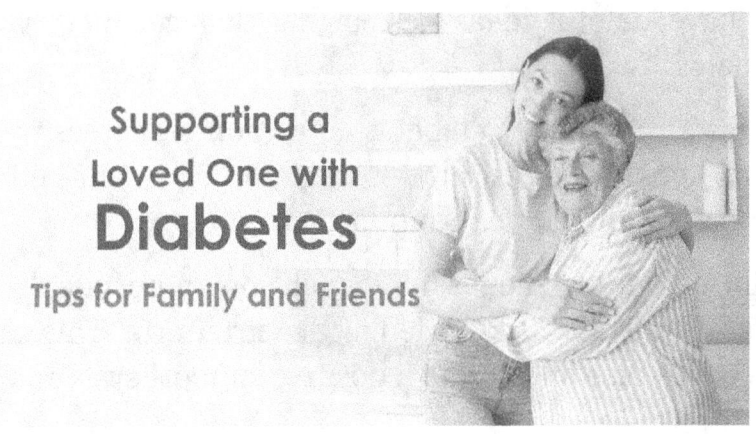

- Educate them about diabetes: Start by teaching your family and friends about diabetes, its symptoms, and how it affects your body. This will help them understand what you're going through and why certain behaviors are important for your health.

- Share your diagnosis: Be open and honest about your diabetes diagnosis and how it affects your daily life. Share your experiences, challenges, and successes with your loved ones.

- Involve them in your care plan: Encourage your family and friends to be part of your care plan by attending doctor's appointments, helping with medication reminders, or joining you for exercise sessions.

- Ask for support: Don't be afraid to ask for help when you need it. Whether it's help with grocery shopping, meal prep, or emotional support, your loved ones can be a valuable resource.

- Make healthy choices together: Encourage your family and friends to make healthy lifestyle choices with you, such as eating a balanced diet, exercising regularly, and getting enough sleep.

- Create a support network: Consider forming a support network with your family and friends, where you can share your experiences, ask for advice, and offer support to one another.

- Celebrate milestones: Celebrate your successes, no matter how small, with your loved ones. This can help motivate you to continue making healthy choices and provide a sense of accomplishment.

- Be open to feedback: Be open to feedback and suggestions from your loved ones. They may have helpful ideas or insights that can help you better manage your diabetes.

- Offer education and resources: Share diabetes education resources with your loved ones, such as books, articles, or websites, to help them better understand the condition and how they can support you.

- Show appreciation: Show your loved ones how much you appreciate their support by expressing gratitude and acknowledging their efforts. This can help strengthen your relationships and create a positive support system.

Remember, involving your family and friends in your diabetes self-care routine can help you feel less alone and more supported in your journey. By working together, you can create a supportive network that can help you manage your diabetes and improve your health and well-being.

Explain the science of diabetes.

Diabetes is a complex disease that is influenced by a combination of genetic, environmental, and lifestyle factors. Here are some of the key scientific concepts related to diabetes:

- Insulin and glucagon: Insulin and glucagon are two hormones that play a critical role in regulating blood sugar levels. Insulin is produced by the pancreas and helps to lower blood sugar levels by facilitating the uptake of glucose by cells. Glucagon, on the other hand, is produced by the pancreas and helps to raise blood sugar levels by stimulating the release of glucose from stored glycogen.

- Insulin resistance: Insulin resistance is a condition in which the body's

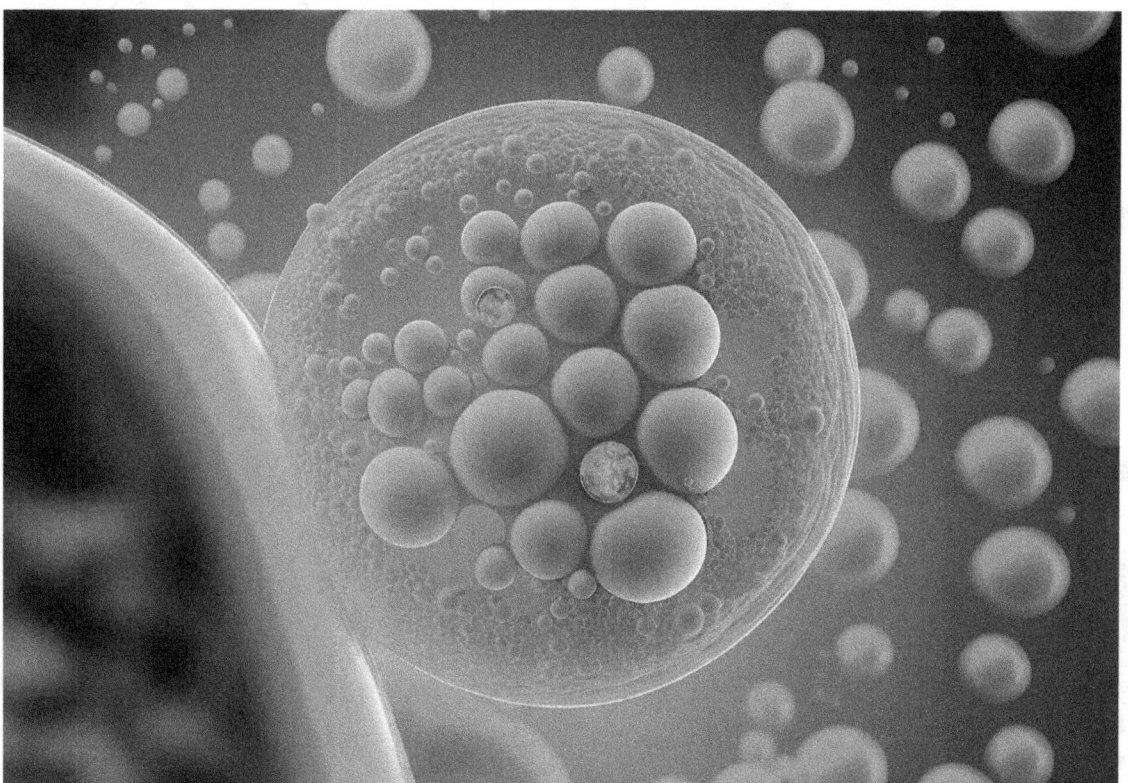

cells become less responsive to insulin, making it harder for glucose to enter the cells. This can lead to high blood sugar levels and is a hallmark of type 2 diabetes.

- Beta cells: Beta cells are the cells in the pancreas that produce insulin. In people with type 1 diabetes, the beta cells are destroyed by the immune system, leading to a complete lack of insulin production.

- Glucose metabolism: Glucose metabolism refers to the process by which the body uses glucose for energy. Glucose is broken down into smaller molecules, such as pyruvate, which can be used by cells for energy production.

- Glycogen: Glycogen is a complex carbohydrate that is stored in the liver and muscles. It is broken down into glucose and released into the bloodstream when the body needs energy.

- Blood sugar regulation: Blood sugar regulation refers to the mechanisms by which the body regulates blood sugar levels. This is achieved through a complex interplay of hormones, including insulin, glucagon, and glucose.

- Type 1 diabetes: Type 1 diabetes is an autoimmune disease in which the immune system attacks and destroys the beta cells in the pancreas, leading to a complete lack of insulin production.

- Type 2 diabetes: Type 2 diabetes is a metabolic disorder that is characterized by insulin resistance, high blood sugar levels, and high levels of insulin. It is often associated with obesity, physical inactivity, and a high-carbohydrate diet.

- Gestational diabetes: Gestational diabetes is a type of diabetes that occurs during pregnancy. It is caused by hormonal changes and insulin resistance, and can lead to complications for both the mother and the baby.

- LADA (latent autoimmune diabetes in adults): LADA is a form of diabetes that is characterized by a slow progression from insulin resistance to a complete loss of insulin production. It is often misdiagnosed as type 2 diabetes.

1 - MODY (maturity-onset diabetes of the young): MODY is a rare form of diabetes that is caused by genetic mutations that affect insulin production. It is characterized by high blood sugar levels and a lack of insulin production.

1 - Secondary diabetes: Secondary diabetes refers to diabetes that develops as a result of another medical condition or treatment, such as pancreatitis, pancreatic surgery, or certain medications.

1 - Monogenic diabetes: Monogenic diabetes refers to diabetes that is caused by a single genetic mutation. It can be diagnosed in children and young adults and is often characterized by a high risk of developing complications.

1 - Polygenic diabetes: Polygenic diabetes refers to diabetes that is caused by multiple genetic mutations. It is more common than monogenic diabetes and is often associated with a family history of diabetes.

1 - Epigenetic diabetes: Epigenetic diabetes refers to diabetes that is caused by changes in gene expression that do not involve a change in the DNA sequence. It is often associated with environmental factors, such as diet and lifestyle.

These are just a few of the many scientific concepts related to diabetes. Understanding these concepts can help individuals with diabetes better manage their condition and improve their quality of life.

Can you explain more about the differences between type 1 and type 2 diabetes?

Type 1 and type 2 diabetes are two distinct forms of diabetes mellitus, a disease characterized by high blood sugar levels. Here are some key differences between the two types:

 - Cause: Type 1 diabetes is an autoimmune disease, meaning that the body's immune system mistakenly attacks and destroys the insulin-producing beta cells in the pancreas, resulting in a complete deficiency of insulin production. Type 2 diabetes, on the other hand, is caused by a combination of insulin resistance (when the body's cells become less

DIABETES MELLITUS
TYPE 1 VS TYPE 2

TYPE 1 DIABETES	TYPE 2 DIABETES
• Occurs when the pancreas is unable to produce enough insulin • Tends to develop at a young age • Cannot be prevented • Require insulin therapy	• Occurs due to insulin resistance (i.e. when the body does not respond well to insulin) • Tends to develop at an older age • Can be prevented with lifestyle changes • Can be managed with lifestyle modifications alone if diagnosed early

• Both share symptoms of frequent urination, increased thirst, extreme hunger, unintentional weight loss, fatigue, blurry vision, sores or wounds that heal slowly, and numbness and tingling sensation in hands and feet.

• Both can benefit from lifestyle modifications such as a healthy diet, physical activity, blood sugar level monitoring, and management of stress and other existing health conditions.

responsive to insulin) and impaired insulin secretion.

- Age of onset: Type 1 diabetes typically develops in childhood or adolescence, while type 2 diabetes typically develops in adulthood, although it can also occur in children and adolescents.

- Insulin production: People with type 1 diabetes produce little to no insulin, while people with type 2 diabetes produce insulin, but their bodies are unable to use it effectively.

- Symptoms: The symptoms of type 1 diabetes can be sudden and severe, including increased thirst and urination, weight loss, fatigue, and blurred vision. Type 2 diabetes symptoms are often milder and may develop gradually over time, including increased thirst and urination, fatigue, and blurred vision.

- Treatment: Type 1 diabetes is typically treated with insulin injections or an insulin pump, which delivers insulin directly into the body. Type 2 diabetes is often treated with lifestyle changes, such as a healthy diet and regular exercise, as well as medications that help the body use insulin more effectively.

- Diet: People with type 1 diabetes need to follow a strict diet that is low in sugar, salt, and fat, and high in fiber and protein. People with type 2 diabetes may need to make similar dietary changes, but the specific recommendations may vary depending on the individual.

- Lifestyle: Both type 1 and type 2 diabetes require regular monitoring of blood sugar levels, but people with type 1 diabetes may need to check their blood sugar more frequently, as they may need to adjust their insulin doses more often.

- Complications: Both type 1 and type 2 diabetes can lead to complications such as nerve damage, kidney damage, and vision problems, but these complications are more likely to occur in people with type 2 diabetes, especially if their condition is not well-managed.

Keep in mind that while these are some of the main differences between type 1 and type 2 diabetes, there can be some overlap between the two conditions, and individuals may have characteristics of both types. A healthcare professional can help determine the specific type of diabetes and develop an appropriate treatment plan.

How can someone determine if they have type 1 or type 2 diabetes?

There are several ways to determine whether someone has type 1 or type 2 diabetes. Here are some of the common methods:

- Blood tests: A healthcare provider may perform blood tests to check for the levels of glucose, hemoglobin A1c (HbA1c), and antibodies (proteins produced by the immune system) in the blood. Type 1 diabetes is characterized by high levels of glucose and HbA1c, and the presence of antibodies against insulin or glutamic acid decarboxylase (GAD), which are enzymes produced by the pancreas. Type 2 diabetes, on the other hand, is characterized by high levels of glucose and HbA1c, but low levels of insulin and absence of antibodies.

- Clinical presentation: The symptoms of type 1 and type 2 diabetes can be different. Type 1 diabetes often presents with sudden and severe symptoms, such as increased thirst and urination, weight loss, fatigue, and blurred vision. Type 2 diabetes, on the other hand, may present with milder symptoms, such as increased thirst and urination, fatigue, and blurred vision, which may develop gradually over time.

- Medical history: A healthcare provider may ask questions about the patient's medical history, such as whether they have a family history of diabetes, whether they have had any previous episodes of hyperglycemia (high blood sugar), or whether they have any other health conditions that may be related to diabetes.

- Physical examination: A healthcare provider may perform a physical examination to look for any signs of diabetes, such as skin changes, nerve damage, or signs of kidney damage.

- Glucose tolerance test: A healthcare provider may perform a glucose tolerance test to determine how well the patient's body responds to glucose. In this test, the patient is given a drink containing a certain amount of glucose, and their blood sugar levels are measured afterward.

- Insulin tolerance test: A healthcare provider may perform an insulin tolerance test to determine how well the patient's body responds to insulin. In this test, the patient is given a small dose of insulin, and their blood sugar levels are measured afterward.

Consider that these tests are not definitive, and a healthcare provider may use a combination of these methods to make a diagnosis. Additionally, some people may have characteristics of both type 1 and type 2 diabetes, and may be diagnosed with a condition called latent autoimmune diabetes in adults (LADA) or double diabetes.

Can you explain more about latent autoimmune diabetes in adults (LADA) and double diabetes?

Latent autoimmune diabetes in adults (LADA) is a form of diabetes that is characterized by the slow progression from insulin resistance to a complete loss of insulin production. It is often referred to as "double diabetes" because it involves both insulin resistance (like type 2 diabetes) and autoimmune destruction of the insulin-producing beta cells (like type 1 diabetes).

LADA typically affects adults over the age of 30, and it is more common in women than men. It often presents with symptoms similar to type 2 diabetes, such as high blood sugar levels, increased thirst and urination, and blurred vision. However, LADA also involves the autoimmune destruction of beta cells, which can lead to a complete loss of insulin production over time.

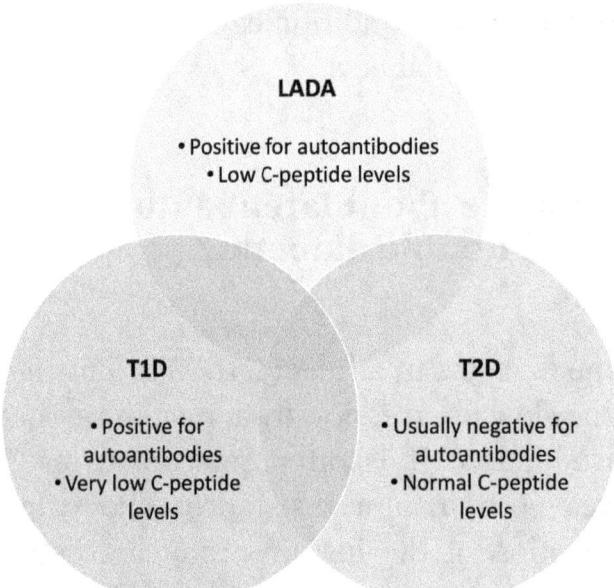

The exact cause of LADA is not fully understood, but it is thought to involve a combination of genetic and environmental factors. It is believed that certain genetic mutations may increase the risk of developing LADA, and exposure to certain environmental triggers, such as viral infections or stress, may also play a role.

Double diabetes refers to the presence of both insulin resistance (like type 2 diabetes) and autoimmune destruction of the insulin-producing beta cells (like type 1 diabetes). This can occur in people with LADA, as well as in some people with type 2 diabetes who develop autoantibodies against their own insulin-producing beta cells.

The diagnosis of LADA and double diabetes can be challenging, as the symptoms and laboratory test results may be similar to those of type 2 diabetes. However, certain tests, such as the presence of autoantibodies against insulin or glutamic acid decarboxylase (GAD), can help to distinguish between the different types of diabetes.

Treatment for LADA and double diabetes typically involves a combination of medications and lifestyle modifications. Insulin therapy may be necessary to manage blood sugar levels, and medications such as metformin or sulfonylureas may be used to improve insulin sensitivity. Lifestyle modifications, such as a healthy diet and regular exercise, can also help to manage blood sugar levels and improve health.

LADA and double diabetes are forms of diabetes that involve both insulin resistance and autoimmune destruction of the insulin-producing beta cells. While the exact cause of LADA is not fully understood, it is believed to involve a combination of genetic and environmental factors. Diagnosis and treatment of LADA and double diabetes can be challenging, but a combination of medications and lifestyle modifications can help to manage blood sugar levels and improve health.

Can you explain the difference between LADA and type 2 diabetes?

LADA (latent autoimmune diabetes in adults) and type 2 diabetes are both forms of diabetes, but they have some key differences.

Type 2 diabetes is a metabolic disorder that is characterized by insulin resistance, which means that the body's cells become less responsive to insulin, a hormone produced by the pancreas that regulates blood sugar levels. As a result, the body produces more insulin to try to keep blood sugar levels under control, but eventually, the pancreas cannot keep up with the demand, and blood sugar levels rise. Type 2 diabetes is often associated with obesity, physical inactivity, and a diet high in sugar and unhealthy fats.

LADA, on the other hand, is a form of diabetes that is characterized by a slow progression from insulin resistance to a complete loss of insulin production. It is often referred to as "double diabetes" because it involves both insulin resistance (like type 2 diabetes) and autoimmune destruction of the insulin-producing beta cells (like type 1 diabetes). LADA typically affects adults over the age of 30, and it is more common in women than men.

The main difference between LADA and type 2 diabetes is the underlying cause of the condition. Type 2 diabetes is caused by a combination of insulin resistance and impaired insulin secretion, while LADA is caused by an autoimmune response that leads to the destruction of the insulin-producing beta cells.

Another key difference is the rate at which the disease progresses. Type 2 diabetes typically progresses slowly over time, while LADA can progress more quickly, often over a period of months or years.

In terms of symptoms, both conditions can cause high blood sugar levels, increased thirst and urination, and blurred vision. However, LADA may also cause weight loss, fatigue, and nausea, which are not typically seen in type 2 diabetes.

While both LADA and type 2 diabetes are forms of diabetes, they have different underlying causes, rates of progression, and symptoms. LADA is an autoimmune condition that involves the destruction of insulin-producing beta cells, while type 2 diabetes is a metabolic disorder caused by insulin resistance and impaired insulin secretion.

Are there any specific risk factors for developing LADA?

Yes, there are several risk factors that have been linked to the development of LADA. Here are some of the most well-established risk factors:

- Genetics: LADA is more common in people with a family history of type 1 diabetes, and certain genetic variants have been identified that increase the risk of developing the condition.

- Autoimmune thyroiditis: LADA is often associated with autoimmune thyroiditis, a condition in which the immune system attacks the thyroid gland. People with autoimmune thyroiditis are at increased risk of developing LADA.

	T1D	'LADA'	T2D	MODY
Typical Age of Onset	All Ages	Usually Age >30	Adults	Usually Age <25
% of all Diabetes	10%	10%	75%	5%
Typical BMI	Mostly Normal or Thin	Mostly Normal or Overweight	Mostly Overweight or Obese	Mostly normal
Ethnicity	All	All	All	All
Progression to insulin Dependence	Fast (Days/Week)	Latent (Months/Years)	Slow (Years)	Depends on MODY type
Insulin Resistance	Mostly no; ~10% ,yes	Some	Yes	Depends on MODY type
Presence of Autoantibodies	Yes (ICA, IA2, GAD65, IAA)	Yes (mostly GAD65), Some not	Some	No
T cell Reponses to islet proteins	Yes	Yes	No	No
Insulin/ C-peptides Level at diagnosis	Undectable or extermly low	Low	Normal to High	Normal
Ketoacidosis	Yes	Yes, many not all	Rare	Rare
Insulin Secretion	Low/null	Varies	Varies	Varies
Islet Inflammation	Chronic Inflammation	Chronic Inflammation	Chronic Inflammation	None
HLA Link	High	Low	None	None
TCF7L2 Link	None	In some pop'n, stronger link than T2D	?5%	None
Other Genes Involved	PTPN22; INS; CTLA4; CCR5; FOXP3;CLEC16a HNF1A; IL2RA; IL6; ITPR3; OAS1; SUMO4	PTPN22; INS	PPARG; JAZF1; KCNJ11; NOTCH2; WFS1; IGF2BP2; FTO; SLC30A8; HHEX	HNF4A; GCK; HNF1A; IPF1; HNF1B; NEUROD1
Early Treatment	Insulin required, diet & exercise helpful	Non-Insulin or insulin, diet & exercise helpful	Non-Insulin, diet & increased activity	Gene Specific
Late Treatment	Insulin, diet, exercise	Insulin, pills, diet, exercise	Insulin, pills, diet, exercise	Gene Specific

- Other autoimmune conditions: People with other autoimmune conditions, such as rheumatoid arthritis, lupus, or psoriasis, are at increased risk of developing LADA.

- Obesity: Obesity is a risk factor for LADA, as it can lead to insulin resistance and increase the risk of developing type 2 diabetes.

- Physical inactivity: A sedentary lifestyle can increase the risk of developing LADA, as regular physical activity helps to improve insulin sensitivity.

- Poor diet: A diet high in processed foods, sugar, and saturated fats can increase the risk of developing LADA, as it can contribute to insulin resistance and inflammation.

- Age: LADA is more common in people over the age of 30, and the risk increases with age.

- Ethnicity: LADA is more common in certain ethnic groups, such as Hispanics and African Americans.

- History of gestational diabetes: Women who have had gestational diabetes during pregnancy are at increased risk of developing LADA later in life.

- Polycystic ovary syndrome (PCOS): Women with PCOS are at increased risk of developing LADA, as PCOS is associated with insulin resistance and autoimmune thyroiditis.

Not everyone with these risk factors will develop LADA, and some people without any known risk factors can still develop the condition. If you have any concerns about your risk for LADA, it's a good idea to talk to your doctor about your individual risk factors and any steps you can take to reduce your risk.

Are there any specific tests or screenings I should undergo to assess my risk for LADA?

Yes, there are several tests and screenings that can help assess your risk for LADA. Here are some of the most common ones:

- Fasting blood sugar (FBS) test: This test measures your blood sugar levels after an overnight fast. A result of 100-125 mg/dL is considered impaired fasting glucose (IFG), which can be an early sign of LADA.

- Oral glucose tolerance test (OGTT): This test measures your blood sugar levels after consuming a sugary drink. A result of 140-199 mg/dL indicates impaired glucose tolerance (IGT), which can progress to LADA.

- Hemoglobin A1c (HbA1c) test: This test measures your average blood sugar levels over the past 2-3 months. A result of -7- -4% indicates insulin resistance, which can be a sign of LADA.

- Autoantibody test: This test detects the presence of autoantibodies against pancreatic islet cells, which are a hallmark of LADA. The presence of these autoantibodies can indicate an increased risk of developing LADA.

- Glucagon stimulation test: This test measures your body's response to glucagon, a hormone that raises blood sugar levels. A decreased response to glucagon can indicate impaired glucose tolerance and an increased risk of LADA.

- Insulin tolerance test: This test measures your body's response to insulin, a hormone that lowers blood sugar levels. A decreased response to insulin can indicate insulin resistance and an increased risk of LADA.

- Genetic testing: Genetic testing can identify genetic variants that increase the risk of developing LADA. However, genetic testing is not yet widely available for LADA, and its clinical usefulness is still being studied.

Keep in mind that these tests are not definitive and may not accurately predict the development of LADA in all individuals. However, they can provide valuable information to help healthcare providers assess an individual's risk and make informed decisions about their care.

If you have any concerns about your risk for LADA, you need to discuss them with your healthcare provider. They can help determine whether you should undergo any of these tests and develop a plan to manage your risk factors.

The role of technology in managing diabetes

Technology has played a significant role in the management of diabetes, providing various tools and resources to help individuals with diabetes monitor and control their condition. Here are some ways technology has impacted diabetes management:

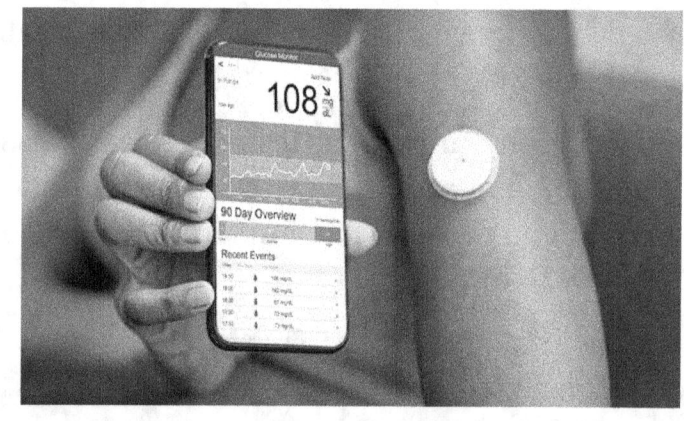

   - Glucose monitoring: Continuous glucose monitoring (CGM) systems, which measure glucose levels throughout the day and night, have become more common. These systems provide real-time glucose data, allowing individuals to make informed decisions about their diet, exercise, and medication.

- Insulin delivery: Insulin pumps, which deliver insulin directly into the body, have become more advanced, allowing for more precise dosing and better control over blood sugar levels. Some pumps also have built-in CGM systems, providing a more comprehensive picture of glucose levels.

   - Mobile apps: There are numerous mobile apps available that help individuals with diabetes track their glucose levels, medication, and diet. These apps can also provide alerts and reminders to take medication, check glucose levels, and engage in physical activity.

- Telemedicine: Telemedicine has made it easier for individuals with diabetes to consult with healthcare professionals remotely, reducing the need for in-person visits. This can be particularly helpful for those living in rural areas or with mobility issues.

- Artificial intelligence: Artificial intelligence (AI) is being used to develop personalized treatment plans for individuals with diabetes. AI algorithms can analyze data from various sources, such as glucose monitoring systems, medical records, and lifestyle data, to provide tailored recommendations for medication, diet, and exercise.

- Wearable devices: Wearable devices, such as smartwatches and fitness trackers, can monitor physical activity, sleep, and other health metrics. This data can be integrated with glucose monitoring and insulin delivery systems, providing a more comprehensive view of an individual's health.

- Virtual reality: Virtual reality (VR) technology is being explored for its potential to improve diabetes management. VR systems can provide immersive experiences that simulate real-life situations, such as cooking healthy meals or engaging in physical activity, helping individuals with diabetes learn new skills and behaviors.

- 3D printing: 3D printing technology has been used to create customized insulin pumps, glucose sensors, and other diabetes-related devices. These customized devices can provide better fit, comfort, and functionality for individuals with diabetes.

- Big data analytics: The abundance of data generated by diabetes management tools, such as glucose monitoring systems and mobile apps, can be analyzed using big data analytics. This can help healthcare professionals identify patterns and trends in diabetes management, leading to more effective treatment strategies.

- Personalized medicine: The increasing availability of genetic and genomic data has enabled the development of personalized medicine approaches for diabetes management. Genetic testing can help identify individuals at risk of developing diabetes, while genomic data can be used to tailor treatment plans to an individual's unique genetic profile.

Technology has revolutionized diabetes management, providing individuals with more control over their condition and enabling healthcare professionals to deliver more personalized and effective care.

Autoantibody test; Insulin tolerance test; Genetic testing

- Autoantibody test: This test detects the presence of autoantibodies against pancreatic islet cells, which are a hallmark of LADA. The presence of these autoantibodies can indicate an increased risk of developing LADA.

- Insulin tolerance test: This test measures your body's response to insulin, a hormone that lowers blood sugar levels. A decreased response to insulin can indicate insulin resistance and an increased risk of LADA.

Insulin Tolerance Test

Insulin tolerance test is a medical diagnosis process during which insulin is injected into a patient vein to examine,

• Pituitary function

• Adrenal function for other purpose.

An ITT is usually ordered and interpreted by the endocrinologist

- Genetic testing: Genetic testing can identify genetic variants that increase the risk of developing LADA. However, genetic testing is not yet widely available for LADA, and its clinical usefulness is still being studied.

- Oral glucose tolerance test (OGTT): This test measures your body's ability to regulate blood sugar levels after consuming a sugary drink. A failed OGTT can indicate impaired glucose tolerance and an increased risk of LADA.

- Fasting plasma glucose (FPG) test: This test measures your blood sugar levels after an overnight fast. A high FPG level can indicate diabetes or impaired glucose tolerance, which can increase the risk of developing LADA.

- Hemoglobin A1c (HbA1c) test: This test measures your average blood sugar levels over the past 2-3 months. A high HbA1c level can indicate diabetes or impaired glucose tolerance, which can increase the risk of developing LADA.

- Urine test: A urine test can detect the presence of ketones, which are a sign of diabetes. A positive urine test can indicate diabetes or impaired glucose tolerance, which can increase the risk of developing LADA.

Note that these tests are not definitive and may not accurately diagnose LADA in everyone. A healthcare professional will use a combination of these tests, along with medical history and physical examination, to diagnose LADA.

Personalized medicine

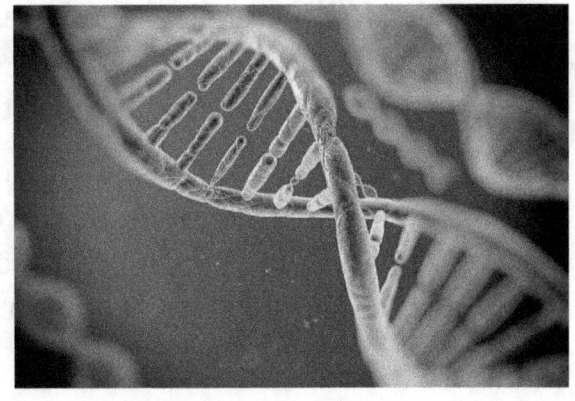

Personalized medicine is an emerging field that aims to tailor medical treatment to an individual's unique genetic, environmental, and lifestyle factors. In the context of diabetes management, personalized medicine approaches can help identify individuals at risk of developing diabetes and tailor treatment plans to an individual's unique genetic profile.

Genetic testing can help identify individuals at risk of developing diabetes by analyzing genetic variants associated with an increased risk of diabetes. For example, genetic tests can identify variants in genes that encode for proteins involved in glucose metabolism, such as the HLA-DQB1*06:02 gene, which is associated with an increased risk of developing type 1 diabetes.

Genomic data can also be used to tailor treatment plans to an individual's unique genetic profile. For example, genomic data can be used to identify genetic variants that affect the metabolism of certain medications, such as metformin, a commonly used medication for type 2 diabetes. By identifying genetic variants that affect metformin metabolism, healthcare providers can tailor the dosage and timing of metformin treatment to an individual's unique genetic profile, which can improve treatment outcomes and reduce the risk of adverse effects.

In addition to genetic testing and genomic data, other personalized medicine approaches for diabetes management include:

 - Precision medicine: This approach involves tailoring medical treatment to an individual's unique genetic, environmental, and lifestyle factors. Precision medicine can help identify the most effective treatment for an individual based on their unique genetic profile.

 - Pharmacogenomics: This approach involves using genomic data to predict an individual's response to certain medications. By identifying genetic variants that affect drug metabolism and response, healthcare providers can tailor medication treatment to an individual's unique genetic profile.

 - Nutrigenomics: This approach involves using genomic data to personalize nutrition recommendations based on an individual's unique genetic profile. By identifying genetic variants that affect nutrient metabolism and response, healthcare providers can tailor nutrition recommendations to an individual's unique genetic needs.

- Microbiome analysis: This approach involves analyzing the genetic material of the microorganisms that live in and on the human body. By identifying the unique genetic profile of an individual's microbiome, healthcare providers can tailor treatment plans to an individual's unique microbial community.

Personalized medicine approaches for diabetes management offer promising opportunities for improving treatment outcomes and reducing the risk of complications associated with diabetes. By tailoring treatment plans to an individual's unique genetic, environmental, and lifestyle factors, healthcare providers can provide more effective and targeted care for individuals with diabetes.

What are some potential benefits of tailoring nutrition recommendations based on an individual's genetic profile?

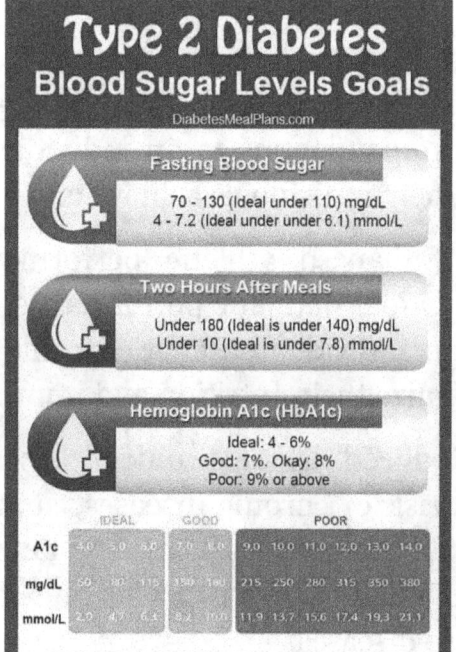

Tailoring nutrition recommendations based on an individual's genetic profile can have several potential benefits, including:

- Improved nutrient absorption and utilization: Genetic variations can affect the way the body absorbs and utilizes nutrients. By tailoring nutrition recommendations to an individual's genetic profile, healthcare providers can ensure that the individual is getting the nutrients they need in the most effective way possible.

- Increased personalization: Genetic testing can provide valuable insights into an individual's unique genetic makeup, which can be used to create personalized nutrition recommendations that are tailored to their specific needs.

- Enhanced health outcomes: By tailoring nutrition recommendations to an individual's genetic profile, healthcare providers can help prevent or manage certain health conditions, such as nutrient deficiencies, that may be more common in certain populations or families.

- Reduced risk of adverse reactions: Genetic variations can also affect the way the body responds to certain foods or nutrients. By tailoring nutrition recommendations to an individual's genetic profile, healthcare providers can reduce the risk of adverse reactions, such as food allergies or intolerances.

- Improved weight management: Genetic variations can affect an individual's metabolism and weight management. By tailoring nutrition recommendations to an individual's genetic profile, healthcare providers can help individuals achieve and maintain a healthy weight.

- Enhanced athletic performance: Genetic variations can affect an individual's athletic performance. By tailoring nutrition recommendations to an individual's genetic profile, healthcare providers can help athletes optimize their nutrition and improve their performance.

- Reduced risk of chronic diseases: Certain genetic variations can increase the risk of chronic diseases, such as heart disease, type 2 diabetes, and certain types of cancer. By tailoring nutrition recommendations to an individual's genetic profile, healthcare providers can reduce the risk of these diseases.

- Improved health: By tailoring nutrition recommendations to an individual's genetic profile, healthcare providers can help individuals achieve optimal health and well-being.

While genetic testing can provide valuable insights into an individual's genetic makeup, it's not a definitive predictor of health outcomes. Other factors, such as lifestyle, environment, and diet, also play a significant role in determining an individual's health.

Can genetic testing accurately predict an individual's nutrient absorption and utilization? How can healthcare providers determine the most effective nutrition recommendations based on an individual's genetic profile? What are some other factors besides genetics that can influence an individual's health outcomes?

Genetic testing can provide some information about an individual's nutrient absorption and utilization, but it is not always accurate. The accuracy of genetic testing for nutrient absorption and utilization depends on several factors, including the type of genetic test, the quality of the test, and the individual's genetic background.

There are several types of genetic tests that can be used to predict nutrient absorption and utilization, including:

 - Genome-wide association studies (GWAS): These tests look for genetic variations associated with specific nutrient absorption and utilization.

 - Whole-genome sequencing: This test provides a comprehensive view of an individual's genetic makeup, including variations that may affect nutrient absorption and utilization.

 - Targeted genetic tests: These tests focus on specific genes or genetic variations that are known to affect nutrient absorption and utilization.

However, it is important to note that genetic testing is only one factor that can influence nutrient absorption and utilization. Other factors, such as lifestyle, diet, and environmental factors, can also play a significant role.

Healthcare providers can determine the most effective nutrition recommendations based on an individual's genetic profile by considering several factors, including:

- Genetic variations: Healthcare providers can use genetic testing to identify genetic variations that may affect nutrient absorption and utilization.

- Dietary patterns: Healthcare providers can assess an individual's dietary patterns and identify potential nutrient deficiencies or excesses.

- Lifestyle factors: Lifestyle factors, such as physical activity level, smoking status, and alcohol consumption, can also influence nutrient absorption and utilization.

- Medical history: Healthcare providers can consider an individual's medical history, including any previous nutrient deficiencies or health conditions, when making nutrition recommendations.

- Nutrient levels: Healthcare providers can measure an individual's nutrient levels, such as vitamin D or iron, to determine if they are deficient or excessive.

Other factors besides genetics that can influence an individual's health outcomes include:

- Lifestyle factors: Lifestyle factors, such as physical activity level, smoking status, and alcohol consumption, can significantly impact health outcomes.

- Environmental factors: Exposure to pollutants, radiation, and other environmental toxins can increase the risk of certain health conditions.

- Dietary patterns: A healthy diet rich in fruits, vegetables, whole grains, and lean proteins can help prevent chronic diseases.

- Stress levels: Chronic stress can increase the risk of mental health conditions, such as depression and anxiety, and can also impact physical health.

- Social support: A strong social support network can help individuals cope with stress and improve their health and well-being.

- Socioeconomic factors: Socioeconomic factors, such as income and education level, can impact access to healthcare and healthy food options, which can ultimately influence health outcomes.

- Cultural factors: Cultural beliefs and practices can influence health behaviors and health outcomes.

- Access to healthcare: Access to healthcare, including preventive care and treatment, can significantly impact health outcomes.

- Age and gender: Age and gender can impact health outcomes, with certain health conditions being more common in certain age groups or genders.

◖ BLOOD SUGAR LEVEL ◗

	A1C TEST	FASTING BLOOD SUGAR TEST	GLUCOSE TOLERANCE TEST
DIABETES	6.5% or above	126 mg/dL or above	200 mg/dL or above
PREDIABETES	5.7-6.4%	100-125 mg/dL	140-199 mg/dL
NORMAL	Below 5.7%	99 mg/dL or below	140 mg/dL or below

Genetic testing can provide some information about an individual's nutrient absorption and utilization, but it is only one factor that healthcare providers should consider when making nutrition recommendations. Other factors, such as lifestyle, diet, and environmental factors, can also play a significant role in determining an individual's health outcomes.

BLOOD SUGAR TRACKER

BLOOD SUGAR TRACKER

DATE	TIME	LEVEL	NOTES	FASTING	EXERCISE	< 20 Carbs	> 20 Carbs	ILLNESS
				○	○	○	○	○
				○	○	○	○	○
				○	○	○	○	○
				○	○	○	○	○
				○	○	○	○	○
				○	○	○	○	○
				○	○	○	○	○
				○	○	○	○	○
				○	○	○	○	○
				○	○	○	○	○
				○	○	○	○	○
				○	○	○	○	○
				○	○	○	○	○
				○	○	○	○	○
				○	○	○	○	○
				○	○	○	○	○
				○	○	○	○	○
				○	○	○	○	○
				○	○	○	○	○

MEAL PLANNER

Diabetes Meal Planner							
Lorem ipsum dolor sit amet, consectetuer adipiscing elit, sed diam nonum Lorem ipsum dolor sit amet, consectetuer adipiscing elit, sed diam nonum.							
*	MON	TUE	WED	THU	FRI	SAT	SUN
BREAKFAST							
LUNCH							
DINNER							
SNACKS							

DISCLAIMER

Seek professional medical advice.

The information contained in this book is not intended to be used as medical advice. The book is intended for educational purposes only and should not be used to diagnose, treat, cure, or prevent any disease. If you have diabetes or are at risk of developing diabetes, it is important to consult with a qualified healthcare professional, such as a diabetes specialist, to receive personalized medical advice and treatment. The information in this book should not be used as a substitute for professional medical advice, diagnosis, or treatment. Always consult with a qualified healthcare professional before making any changes to your diet, exercise, or medication regimen. The author and publisher of this book disclaim any liability or responsibility for any adverse effects or consequences resulting from the use of the information contained in this book.

NOTES

NOTES

NOTES

NOTES

NOTES

NOTES

NOTES

NOTES

NOTES

NOTES

DIABETES SELF-CARE SKILLS

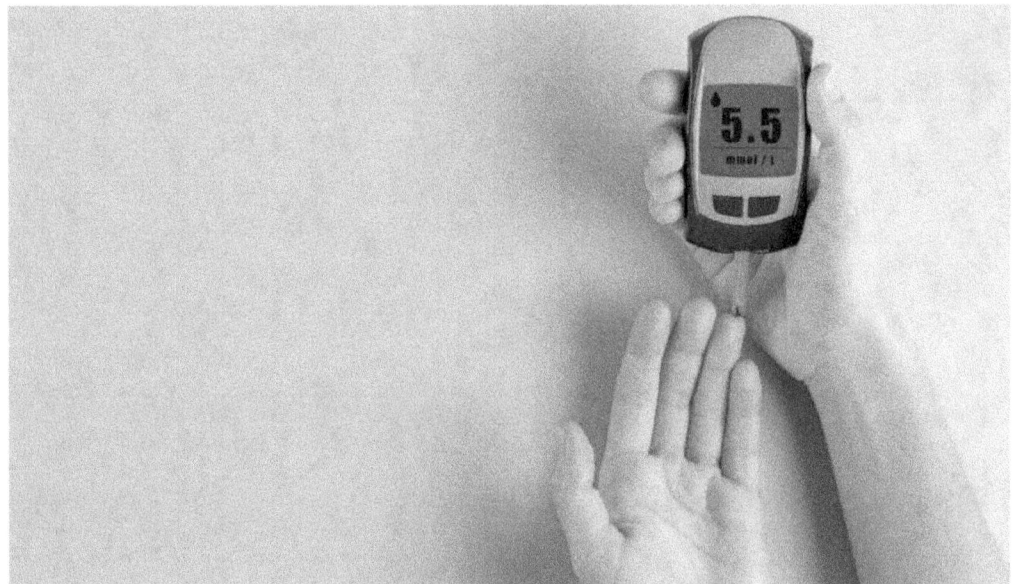

Table of Contents

What is Diabetes?

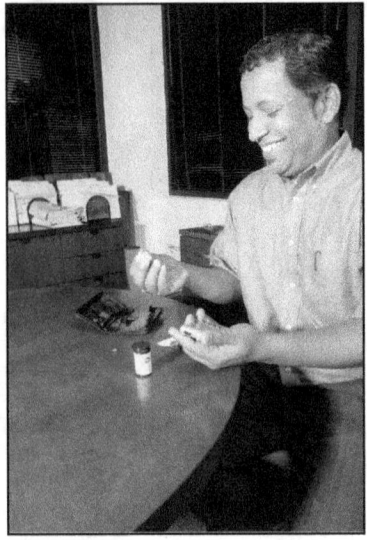

Before you had diabetes, your body controlled the sugar in your blood on its own. You did not even have to think about it. Your body used insulin to get you the energy you needed. This system worked perfectly all day, every day.

Things are different now. Left untreated, your diabetes could increase your blood sugars to the point of damage to your body.

Diabetes is a disease in which the body does not produce or properly use insulin. Insulin is a hormone that is needed to change carbohydrates into energy needed for daily life. The cause of diabetes continues to be a mystery, although both genetics and environmental factors such as obesity and lack of exercise appear to play roles.

Diabetes can be diagnosed using several different tests.
- A random blood sugar of 200 or greater
- A fasting blood sugar of 126 or greater
- An Oral Glucose Tolerance test of 200 or greater
- HgbA1C > 6.5%

Type 1 Diabetes
People with type 1 make little or no insulin. They must take insulin in order to survive. This type usually happens in young people, but can happen at any age.

Symptoms of Type 1
- need to urinate often
- increase thirst
- increase in hunger
- loss of weight without trying to lose
- weakness or tiredness

What is Diabetes?

Type 2 Diabetes

People with type 2 still make insulin. Their bodies may not make enough insulin or their cells are resistant to the insulin they do make. It is most often found after the age of forty, but can happen at any age. Many people with type 2 are overweight.

Symptoms of Type 2
- need to urinate often
- increase thirst
- increase in hunger
- tiredness
- blurred vision
- dry, itchy skin
- frequent infections
- slow healing cuts or sores

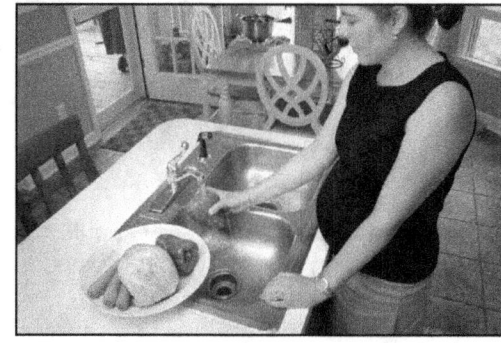

Gestational Diabetes

Gestational diabetes is a type of diabetes that occurs only in pregnancy and usually disappears after the birth of the baby. It is usually detected at 24 to 28 weeks of pregnancy. In all pregnancies, the placenta creates hormones that work against the action of insulin, reducing its effectiveness. In most women, the pancreas is able to make extra insulin to overcome insulin resistance. If your pancreas is unable to make enough insulin and your blood sugar remains too high, this is known as gestational diabetes.

Who is likely to have it?
- family history of diabetes
- previous birth of a very large baby
- are overweight
- earlier pregnancy with gestational diabetes
- too much amniotic fluid
- older than 25 years

Pre-diabetes

The term "borderline diabetes" has been replaced with the more appropriate term of pre-diabetes. These individuals have impaired fasting glucose (IFG) and/or impaired glucose tolerance (IGT). They are at a higher risk of developing type 2 diabetes. It is estimated that over 5 years, 30 to 40% of these individuals will develop type 2 diabetes.

IFG (Impaired fasting glucose)
- Fasting blood sugar level between 100 and 125
IGT (Impaired glucose tolerance)
- After meal blood sugar level between 140 and 199

What Happens When We Eat?

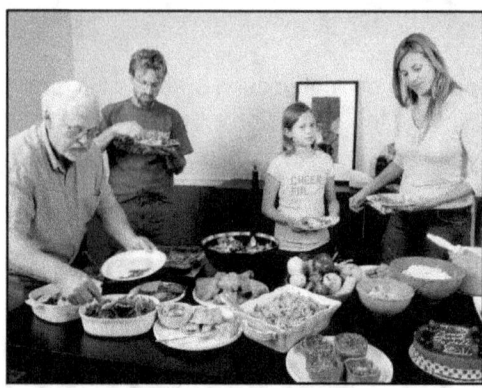

When we eat, all of our foods contain:
- Carbohydrates
- Proteins
- Fats

Carbohydrates are the main source of energy for the body. We all need a certain amount of carbohydrates whether we have diabetes or not. When we eat carbohydrates our bodies take those nutrients and convert them to a form of sugar called glucose that we use for energy. So, trying to control your blood sugar by not eating carbohydrates is not good for your body.

Let's look at the process of what should happen in your body when you eat. Seeing the normal process of eating will help you better understand what may be happening in your body and why you were diagnosed with diabetes.

Normal Physiology of Eating

Carbohydrate digestion begins as soon we start eating. Enzymes in the mouth start to break down carbohydrates into sugar (glucose) that our body uses for energy. In fact, when someone without diabetes sees or smells food the brain signals the pancreas to release any stored insulin. Insulin is needed to digest carbohydrates. This signaling is called the **first phase response** and most individuals with Type 2 diabetes have lost the first phase response.

Carbohydrates travel from the mouth and travel down the esophagus into the stomach. The carbohydrates continue their change to sugar before entering the small intestine. At this point, the sugar trickles through the wall of the intestines and enters the bloodstream. The pancreas then secretes just the right amount of insulin to match the sugar present in the bloodstream. Insulin is the key that opens the door on our cells so that the sugar from the blood enters the cells where it is used for energy.

In other words, insulin "unlocks" and opens the doors of the cells allowing the sugar to enter and be used for energy. When something in this process fails the result can be a diagnosis of diabetes.

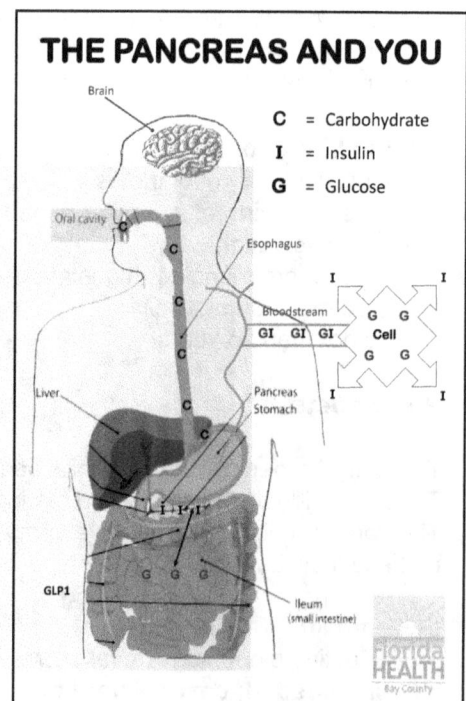

THE PANCREAS AND YOU

C = Carbohydrate
I = Insulin
G = Glucose

Monitoring Blood Sugar

Monitoring your blood sugar can help you to control your blood sugar levels.

Testing your own blood glucose levels is a key to taking charge of your diabetes.

Blood glucose testing can help you understand how food, physical activity, and diabetes medicine affect your glucose levels. Testing can help you make day-to-day choices about how to balance these things. It can also tell you when your glucose is too low or too high so that you can treat these problems.

How to Test your blood sugar

1. Wash your hands with soap and water.
2. Place a needle in the Lancet device (check the depth setting).
3. Insert a strip into your meter (this will turn the machine on).
4. Press the Lancet device on the side of the finger to get a drop of blood.
5. Touch and hold the end of the test strip to the drop of blood. It will "suck up" the blood.
6. Wait for the result.

Possible times to Monitor:

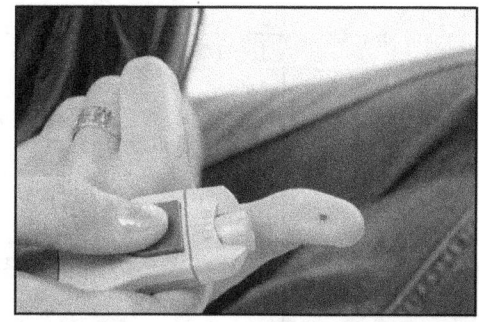

- Fasting
- Bedtime
- Before Meals
- 2 Hours after start of Meals
- Any symptoms of High or Low Blood Sugar
- Before and After Exercise
- During Times of Unusual Stress or Illness
- When Dosing Insulin Based on Blood Sugar

You can develop a schedule where you get to see all the important times with only check 1 to 2 times per day.

Remember monitoring is individual and everyone's schedule will be different….

BLOOD SUGAR GOALS	AACE*	ADA**
Before Eating	70-110	80-130
Two hours after eating	<140	<180
Hemoglobin A1C%	<6.5%	<7.0%

*American Association of Clinical Endocrinologists Guidelines (AACE)
**American Diabetes Association (ADA)

Monitoring Blood Sugar

Day 1	Day 2	Day 3	Day 4	Day 5	Day 6
Date: **Bedtime** Time: Result:	Date: **Fasting** Time: Result:	Date: **Before Lunch** Time: Result: **After Lunch** Time: Result:	Date: **Before Dinner** Time: Result: **After Dinner** Time: Result:	Date: **Before Exercise** Time: Result: **After Exercise** Time: Result:	Date: **Not feeling well or stressed** Time: Result:
Day 7	**Day 8**	**Day 9**	**Day 10**	**Day 11**	**Day 12**
Date: **Before Breakfast** Time: Result: **After Breakfast** Time: Result:	**Take the day off**	Date: **Bedtime** Time: Result:	Date: **Fasting** Time: Result:	Date: **Before Lunch** Time: Result: **After Lunch** Time: Result:	Date: **Before Dinner** Time: Result: **After Dinner** Time: Result:
Day 13	**Day 14**	**Day 15**	**Day 16**	**Day 17**	**Day 18**
Date: **Before Exercise** Time: Result: **After Exericse** Time: Result:	Date: **Not feeling well or stressed** Time: Result:	Date: **Before Breakfast** Time: Result: **After Breakfast** Time: Result:	**Take the day off**	Date: **Bedtime** Time: Result:	Date: **Fasting** Time: Result:
Day 19	**Day 20**	**Day 21**	**Day 22**	**Day 23**	**Day 24**
Date: **Before Lunch** Time: Result: **After Lunch** Time: Result:	Date: **Before Dinner** Time: Result: **After Dinner** Time: Result:	Date: **Before Exericse** Time: Result: **After Exercise** Time: Result:	Date: **Not feeling well or stressed** TIme: Result:	**Take the day off**	Date: **Bedtime** Time: Result:
Day 25	**Day 26**	**Day 27**	**Day 28**	**Day 29**	**Day 30**
Date: **Fasting** Time: Result:	Date: **Before Lunch** Time: Result: **After Lunch** Time: Result:	Date: **Before Dinner** Time: Result: **After Dinner** Time: Result:	Date: **Before Exercise** Time: Result: **After Exericse** Time: Result:	Date: Time: Result:	**Take the day off**

Monitoring Blood Sugar

Hemoglobin A1C is an average blood sugar over the past 3 months. It should be checked every 3 months.

HEMOGLOBIN A1C	LEVEL OF CONTROL	AVERAGE BLOOD GLUCOSE
16.0%		420
15.0%		390
14.0%	POOR TAKE ACTION!	360
13.0%		330
12.0%		300
11.0%		270
10.0%		240
9.5%		225
9.0%		210
8.5%		195
8.0%	FAIR	180
7.5%		165
7.0%		150
6.5%	TARGET	135
6.0%	GOOD	120

Oral Medications & Injectables

Oral medications are used to treat Type 2 diabetes. They generally assist the body to produce more insulin or help the body use the insulin it does make better.

TYPE OF MEDICATION	HOW IT WORKS	WHAT YOU CAN EXPECT	WHAT YOU NEED TO KNOW	HOW MUCH IT WILL COST
Glucotrol (glipizide), Amaryl (flimeperide), Glynase (glyburide), Prandin, Starliz	Makes the pancreas make insulin.	Should be taken with or before the meal.	Can cause low blood sugar, weight gain.	Inexpensive.
Glucophage (metformin)	Keeps liver form dumping glucose.	Take with a meal to prevent stomach upset.	Does not cause low blood sugar, may take up to 3 weeks to lower blood sugar.	Inexpensive (certain dose free at Publix).
Januvia, Onglyza, Tradjenta	Blocks an enzyme that assists with blood sugar control.	Take at anytime, no major side effects.	Does not cause low blood sugar.	Can be expensive depending on insurance.
Inovkana, Farxiga, Jardiance	Increases the output of glucose in the urine.	Take at anytime, may cause UTI or yeast infections.	Does not cause low blood sugar.	Can be expensive depending on insurance.
Actos (piogiltazone), Avandia	Helps your body use insulin.	Take at anytime, can cause weight gain.	Does not cause low blood sugar, watch possible weight gain.	Generic is less expensive.
Byetta, Victoza	Helps your body with insulin production and digestion.	Byetta is taken twice a day, up to an hour before breakfast and supper, Vitoza may be taken at anytime in the day.	Given through an injection, does not cause low blood sugar, can cause nausea and other stomach problems.	Can be expensive depending on insurance.
Bydureon, Tanzeum, Trulicity	Helps your body with insulin production and digestion.	Taken once a week.	Given through an injection, does not cause low blood sugar, can cause nausea and other stomach problems.	Can be expensive depending on insurance.

Insulin

TYPE OF INSULIN	Rapid	Fast	Intermediate	Long	Mixed
BRAND NAME	Humalog, Novolog, Apidra	Humulin R, Novolin R, ReliOn	Humulin N. Novolin N, ReliOn	Lantus, Levermir	Novolog 70/30, Humalog 75/25 & 50/50, Humulin 70/30, Novolin 70/30
WHEN SHOULD YOU TAKE IT?	0-15 min before meal	30 min before meal	Every 12-24 hours.	Same time every day.	Before breakfast and before supper.
HOW LONG DOES IT KEEP WORKING?	3-4 hours	3-6 hours	10-16 hours	20-24 hours	3-24 hours
HOW IS IT PACKAGED?	Vials and pens, safe at room temperature once opened	Vials and pens, safe at room temprea-ture once opened	Vials and pens, safe at room temperature once opened.	Vials and pens, safe at room temperature once opened.	Vials and pens, safe at room temperature once opened.
WHAT DOES IT LOOK LIKE?	Clear	Clear	Cloudy	Clear	Cloudy
SPECIAL CON-SIDERATIONS	Inject immediately before a meal. After meal injection may be beneficial for children or anyone with an unpredictable food intake	May be mixed with intermediate insulin.	Must be mixed before injecting. May be mixed with regular insulin.	Should not be mixed with other insulins. Generally given at beditme, but may be taken at other times. Should be consistent with the time given. One dose may be split into two dose if is is > than 50 units.	Should not be mixed with other insulins. Should be given before meals.
HOW MUCH WILL IT COST?	May be expensive depending on insurance coverage.	Less expensive.	Less expensive.	May be expensive depending on insurance coverage.	Some are less expensive.

Insulin

Administration and Storage

- Keep unused vials/pens refrigerated at 36 to 46 degrees
- Opened vials and pens may be kept at 59 to 86 degrees for one month
- Keep insulin out of direct sunlight
- Cloudiness, discoloration, clumping, or frosting is a sign of decreased potency and should be discarded.
- Insulin should be given into fatty tissue at a 90 degree angle (45 degree angle for a thin person).
- Count to 5 (while needle is still in body) after giving an injection
- Injections may be given in the upper arm, the anterior and lateral aspects of thigh, buttocks, abdomen (with the exception of a 2 inch circle around the navel).
- Rotate the injection sites to decrease the risk of infection
- Abdomen site leads to the most rapid absorption followed by the arms, thighs, and buttocks.

Possible places to give an injection:

- Stomach
- Legs
- Arms
- Top of butt

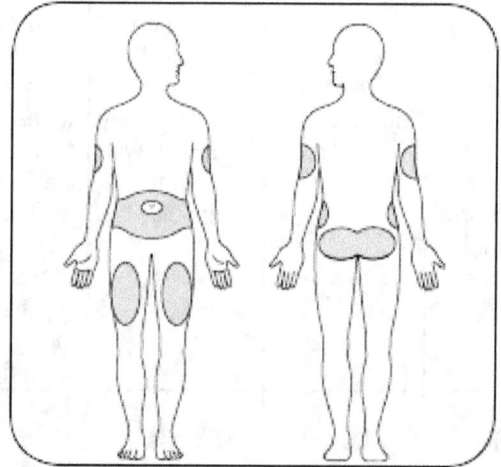

Hypoglycemia

What are the symptoms of hypoglycemia?

The symptoms of hypoglycemia include:

- Shakiness
- Sweating
- Headache
- Seizure
- Sudden moodiness
- Behavior changes
- Difficulty pay attention

- Dizziness
- Hunger
- Pale skin color
- Clumsy/jerky movements
- Confusion
- Tingling sensations around the mouth

How do you know when blood sugar is low?

Hypoglycemia is a blood sugar reading < 70.

- Check your blood glucose whenever you feel any low blood glucose symptoms coming on. After you check and see that your blood glucose level is low, you should treat hypoglycemia quickly.
- If you feel a reaction coming on but cannot check, it's best to treat the reaction rather than wait. Remember this simple rule: When in doubt, treat.

How do you treat hypoglycemia?

Be sure you always carry a fast acting carbohydrate with you.

Use the "Rule of 15" to treat hypoglycemia

1. If your blood glucose is less than 70, have 15 grams of carbohydrates (4 oz juice, 4 glucose tablets, 5 life savers, 15 jelly beans).
2. Wait 15 minutes and recheck your blood glucose.
3. If your blood glucose is still less than 70, take an additional 15 grams of carbohydrates.
4. Wait 15 minutes and recheck blood glucose.
5. Continue this process until blood glucose is greater than 70.
6. If it is close to the time of a meal, eat your meal. If it is not close to the time of a meal, eat a snack.

If you pass out from hypoglycemia, people should:
- NOT inject insulin.
- NOT give you food or fluids.
- NOT put their hands in your mouth.
- Inject glucagon.
- Call for emergency help.

The main causes of low blood sugars are too much medication, too much insulin, not enough food, or skipping meals.

How Food Affects Your Blood Sugar

Many people think that having diabetes means you can't eat your favorite foods. You can still eat the foods you like. It's the amount that counts. Healthy eating habits for diabetes include foods from all major food groups. These foods provide you with the energy and the nutrients you need for good health.

- **Carbohydrates are the only food that directly impacts your blood sugar.**
- Carbs are in foods such as breads, pasta, cereal, beans, potatoes, fruits, fruit juice, yogurt, milk, as well as cakes, pies, cookies, and candy.
- EATING TO MAINTAIN A HEALTHY BLOOD SUGAR
- Balance your carbohydrate intake during the day using the plate method (below).
- Try to not skip meals.
- Eat more non-starchy vegetables.
- Eat less fatty or fried foods.
- When you sit down for a meal, draw an imaginary line through the center of your plate. Draw a line to divide one into two sections.
- ¼ of your plate should be filled with grains or starchy foods such as rice, pasta, potatoes, corn, or peas.
- ¼ of your plate should be lean protein such as meat, fish, or poultry.
- The remaining ½ of your plate should be filled with non starchy vegetables such as lettuce, broccoli, carrots, tomatoes, and etc.
- Add a glass of non-fat milk and a small piece of fruit.

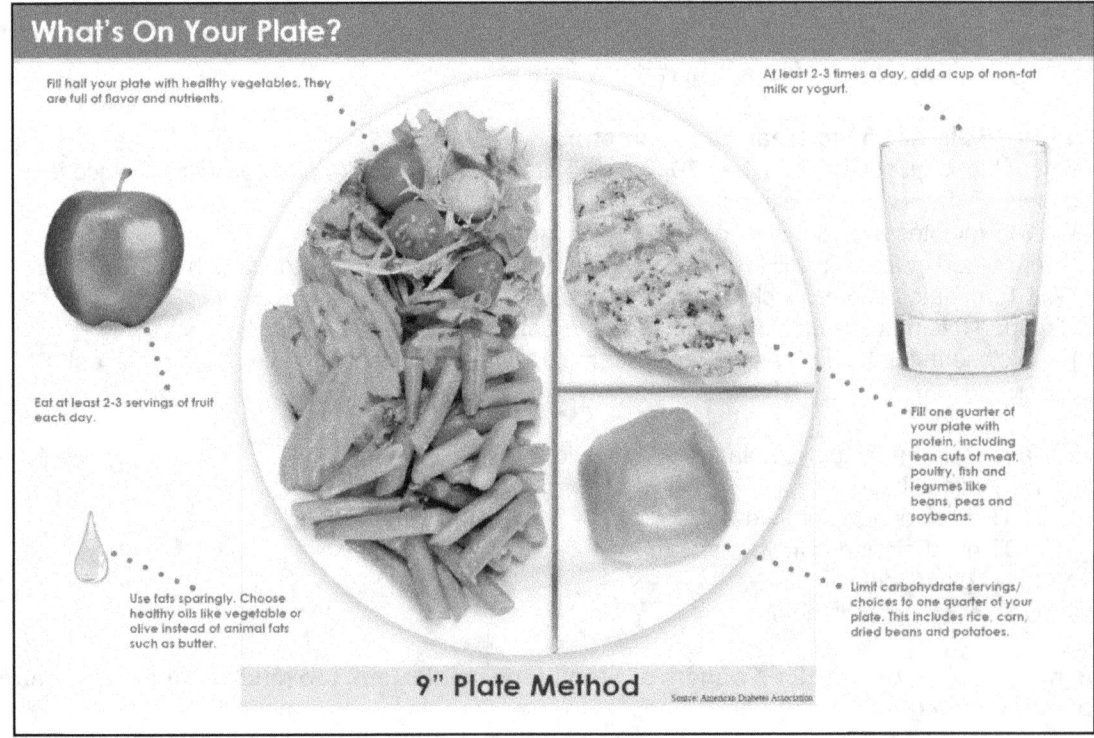

How Food Affects Blood Sugar

MyPlate Food Group	Serving Examples	
Starch/Grains	• 1/2 medium bagel • 1 slice bread • 1/2 English muffin • 1/4 cup cooked pasta or rice • 1- 6 inch tortilla	• 1/2 cup beans • 3/4 cup dry cereal • 4-6 crackers • 1 small potato
Fruit	• 1 medium apple • 1/2 medium banana • 1 cup berries • 1/2 cup grapes • 1 cup melon	• 1 small orange • 1/2 grapefruit • 1 medium pear • 1/2 cup fruit juice
Milk	• 1 cup milk (any type) • 6-8 oz. plain non-fat yogurt • 6-8 oz. light yogurt	
Vegetable	1 cup raw vegetables or 1/2 cup cooked vegetables: • broccoli • cucumber • carrots • cauliflower • celery • green beans • peppers	• 1/2 cup V-8 or tomato juice • greens (kale, collard, mustard) • tomatoes • asparagus • spinach • summer squash • zucchini • lettuce
Protein	• 1 oz. fish • 1 oz. skinless chicken or turkey • 1 oz. lean beef, pork, lamb or veal • 1 oz. low fat cheese	• 1 egg • 1/4 cup egg substitute • 1/4 cup cottage cheese • 2 tbsp. peanut butter
Fats & Oils	• 1 tsp. butter, oil, soft margarine or mayonnaise • 10 peanuts • 6 almonds • 9 cashews • 1 tbsp. cream cheese or salad dressing	• 2 tbsp. light cream chees or light salad dressing • 1 tsp. vegetable oil • 1 slice bacon • 3 tbsp. low fat sour cream • 1/8 of an avocado

How much is a serving of carbohydrate? Each serving below contains 15 grams of carbs.

Examples of one serving:
- 1 slice of bread
- 1 small potato
- 1/2 cup cooked cereal or 3/4 dry cereal flakes
- 1 small tortilla
- 1 small apple

- 1/2 cup juice
- 1/2 grapefruit
- 1 cup low-fat or fat-free yogurt
- 1 cup skim or 1% milk

Sick Day Management

- Drink plenty of fluids.
- Increase blood sugar monitoring. Check blood sugars every 2 to 4 hours.
- Do not stop taking oral medications or insulin. Infection can cause blood sugars to go up.
- Consume some carbohydrates every 3 to 4 hours such as regular jello or soda.

Suggestions of when to give the Doctor a call:

- Experience vomiting and are unable to tolerate fluids.
- Diarrhea for more than 6 hours
- Change in Mental Status
- A pattern of blood sugar levels > 200
- A pattern of blood sugar levels < 70
- Injury to foot or leg
- Low grade fever, < 101.5 degrees
- Any non-healing sores or ulcers
- Urine Ketones

Suggestions of when to seek immediate medical care:

- Vomiting or having diarrhea for more than 6 hours
- Moderate to large amounts of ketones in your urine
- Glucose level > 300 on two readings without response to insulin
- Glucose level > 400
- Severe abdominal pain
- Severe pain anywhere in the body
- Fever > 101.5 degrees
- Unexplained shortness of breath or irregular heartbeat
- Chest pain
- Large sores or ulcers, or cuts penetrating all layers of skin

Resources

Organizations:

American Diabetes Association
www.diabetes.org
1-800-342-2283

Academy of Nutrition and Dietetics
www.eatright.org

Joslin Diabetes Center
www.joslin.org
1-617-309-2400

Online Resources:

- www.doihaveprediabetes.org
- www.dlife.com
- www.diabetescontrolforlife.com
- www.DiabeticLivingOnline.com
- www.diabetesselfmanagement.com
- www.journeyforcontrol.com

Diabetes, Medication, and Food information:

BD Diabetes
www.bd.com/us/diabetes

Cornerstones for Care
www.cornerstones4care.com

Healthy Plate
www.choosemyplate.gov

National Diabetes Education Program
http://ndep.nih.gov
1-301-496-3583

Medication Assistance:

Family Services Agency
114 E. 9th ST
Panama City, FL 32401
850-785-1721

Amylin
1-800-3330-7647

Bayer Corporation
1-800-998-9180

Bristol Myers Squibb
1-800-763-0003

Eli Lilly and Co.
1-800-545-6962

GlaxSmithKline Beecham
1-800-546-0420

Hoechst-Marion-Roussel
1-800-362-7466

Novo Nordisk
1-866-310-7549

Novartis (Starlix)
1-800-277-2254

Pfizer, Inc.
1-800-707-8990

Sanofi-Aventis Pharmaceuticals, Inc.
1-800-446-6267

Needy Meds
www.needsmeds.com

Resources

Apps:

dLife
Backed by the resouces of the #1 diabetes website, offers you access to the most essentials tools you'll need to manage your diabetes on the go.

GoMeals
Makes it easy to access nutritional information, find restaurants and keep track of your food intake.

SparkRecipes
Lets you browse and search more than 190,000 recipes by course, ethincitiy, preparation time, and dietary needs.

Diabetes Tracker
Lets you track your food, blood sugar levels, exericse, blood pressure, weight, medications, and moods- it can all be tracked and put into a report.

Fooducate
Allows you to scan any food product with a UPC to grade your groceries, explain what's really inside each product, create shopping lists, and offers healthier alternatives.

Calorie King
Need a quick and easy way to check calories, carbs, and fat? The CalorieKing Food Database ia America's best and most reliable.

MyPlate
Serves as a reminder to help consumers make helthier food choices with the internet to prompt consumers to think about building a healthy plate.

Lose It!
One of the most popular weight loss apps in the US. It helps you set weight loss goals, establish a daily calorie budget, and enables you to lose weight.

OnTrackDiabetes
Designed to document blood sugar levels, food, A1c, weight and more, then calculates avrages and maintains a record of your history so it's easy to show your doctor how you've been doing.